Copyright 2020 by Shelly Stewart

All rights reserved. No part of this publication may be reproduced, distributed, or transmitted in any form or by any means, including photocopying, recording, or other electronic or mechanical methods, without the prior written permission of the author, except in the case of brief quotations embodied in critical reviews and certain other noncommercial uses permitted by copyright law.

Although the author and publisher have made every effort to ensure that the information in this book was correct at press time, the author and publisher do not assume and hereby disclaim any liability to any party for any loss, damage, or disruption caused by errors or omissions, whether such errors or omissions result from negligence, accident, or any other cause.

By reading this document, the reader agrees that under no circumstances is the author responsible for any losses, direct or indirect, that are incurred as a result of the use of the information contained within this document, including, but not limited to, errors, omissions, or inaccuracies.

CONTENTS

Introduction 6
Chapter 1: What is a Plant-Based Diet? 6
    What is a Vegan Bodybuilding Diet? 6
    Potential Benefits of the Vegan Bodybuilding Diet 7
    The Plant-Based Athlete 7
    Protein and Recovery 8
    How Much Protein is Needed? 9
    Protein Muscle Synthesis 9
Chapter 2: Macros and Micros 10
    Plant-Based Protein Sources 10
    Food to Avoid on a Plant-Based Diet 11
    Macronutrients 11
    Micronutrient Intake 12
Chapter 3: Plant-Based Supplements 14
    Cheat Days 15
    Management and Fitness Goals 15
ESSENTIAL RECIPES 17
    Green Smoothie Bowl 17
    Savory Crepes 18
    Blueberry Waffles 19
    Baked Tofu 20
    Chickpeas Falafel Bowl 21
    Glazed Carrots 22
    Barley & Chickpea Soup 23
    Lentil Soup 24
    Beans & Pasta Stew 25
    Mocha Tofu Pudding 26
BREAKFAST RECIPES 27
    Overnight Porridge 27
    Pumpkin Porridge 28
    Quinoa, Oats, & Seeds Porridge 29
    Barley Porridge 30
    Banana Pancakes 31
    Spinach & Tomato Omelet 32
    Veggie Omelet 33
    Veggie Quiche 34
    Fruity Muffins 35
    Nuts, Seeds, & Coconut Granola 36

HIGH-PROTEIN SNACKS RECIPES 37
- Spiced & Herbed Nuts 37
- Spicy Chickpeas 38
- Nuts & Seeds Squares 39
- Seed Bars 40
- Oatmeal Cookies 41

NUTRIENT-PACKED PROTEIN SALAD RECIPES 42
- Quinoa & Chickpea Salad 42
- Mixed Grain Salad 43
- Rice & Tofu Salad 44
- Kidney Bean & Pomegranate Salad 45
- Bean & Corn Salad 46
- Pasta & Veggie Salad 47
- Chickpea & Veggie Salad 48
- Farro & Veggie Salad 49
- Chickpea & Veggie Salad 50
- Bean & Couscous Salad 51

STAPLE LUNCH RECIPES 52
- Couscous-Stuffed Bell Peppers 52
- Pasta with Asparagus 53
- Black-Eyed Peas Curry 54
- Lentil Falafel Bowls 55
- Buddha Bowl 57
- Vegetarian Taco Bowl 58
- Tofu & Veggie Burgers 59
- Buckwheat Burgers 60
- Stuffed Avocados 61
- Stuffed Sweet Potatoes 62

WHOLE FOOD LUNCH & DINNER RECIPES 63
- Cauliflower with Peas 63
- Burgers with Mushroom Sauce 64
- Rice & Lentil Loaf 66
- Chickpeas with Swiss Chard 68
- Spicy Black Beans 69
- Mixed Bean Soup 70
- Barley & Lentil Stew 71
- Chickpea & Pasta Curry 72
- 3-Bean Chili 73
- Rice Paella 74

GRAINS & BEANS RECIPES 76

- Baked Beans 76
- Chickpeas with Veggies 77
- Beans with Salsa 78
- Bean, Corn, & Salsa Chili 79
- Chili Corn Cane 80
- Beans & Quinoa with Veggies 81
- Lentil Curry 82
- Nut Roast Dinner 83
- Rice & Lentil Casserole 84
- Pasta & Veggie Casserole 85

VEGETABLE RECIPES 86
- Dried Fruit Squash 86
- Banana Curry 87
- Mushroom Curry 88
- 3-Veggie Combo 89
- Beet Soup 90
- Veggie Stew 91
- Tofu with Brussels Sprouts 92
- Tofu with Peas 93
- Carrot Soup with Tempeh 94
- Tempeh with Bell Peppers 95

QUICK ENERGY & RECOVERY SNACKS RECIPES 96
- Date & Seed Bites 96
- Chocolatey Oat Bites 97
- Brownie Bites 98
- Fruity Bites 99
- Energy Bars 100

DRINKS & DESSERT RECIPES 101
- Strawberry Shake 101
- Chocolatey Banana Shake 102
- Fruity Tofu Smoothie 103
- Green Fruity Smoothie 104
- Protein Latte 105
- Chocolatey Bean Mousse 106
- Tofu & Strawberry Mousse 107
- Tofu & Chia Seed Pudding 108
- Banana Brownies 109
- Brown Rice Pudding 110

SAUCES RECIPES 111
- Tofu Mayonnaise 111

  Chickpea Hummus 112
  Peanut Butter Sauce 113
  Tomato Sauce 114
  Mango BBQ Sauce 115
30-Day Meal Plan 116
Cheap Shopping List 118

Introduction
Chapter 1: What is a Plant-Based Diet?

To start with, let's get a clear view of the plant-based diet. This diet, though widely popular, is often confused with a vegetarian diet. The concept is to avoid all animal-sourced food products and rely completely on plant produce. The reasons can vary for each individual. Some may opt for a plant-based diet for its health benefits; others may want to adopt it to save animals—while few others may do so for both such reasons.

What constitutes a plant-based diet? By plant-sourced food, we mean all variety of vegetables, fruits, grains, legumes, lentils, plant oils, seeds, nuts, plant-based milk, grain flours, and vegan cheeses and milk. These products—or the food prepared purely from them—is referred to as vegan or plant-based. In this list, we find that not a single ingredient is purely protein-based. While protein is largely present in most of the plant-sourced products, it is coupled with other macro and micronutrients as well. For athletes and bodybuilders, the concern is how to consume such products while balancing the proportion of these nutrients in the interest of their muscle building. And that concern leads us to the plant-based, vegan bodybuilding diet.

What is a Vegan Bodybuilding Diet?

Every bodybuilder, irrespective of gender, strives to build a strong musculature through heavy training and intensive resistance exercises. And mere exercises can't make much of a difference when there isn't a good diet to support the body changes. Nutrients play a major role in muscle development, and the role of both the macro and the micronutrients cannot be overlooked. Experts believe that for optimal muscle development, about 0.7–1 gram of protein per pound of body weight per day is essential to consume. Keep these values in mind while we make a case for our high protein vegan diet. A bodybuilder must also have a 20% surplus of caloric intake for building and strengthening muscles.

The rise of the plant-based diet has also attracted many athletes and bodybuilders, but many have been skeptical and hesitant to opt for this approach as they were not aware of how a plant-based diet can also be a good source of protein and calories. This particular concern of bodybuilders led many health experts and nutritionists to work extensively on the vegan diet and create high-protein recipes and develop a dietary approach which can specifically meet the needs of the people who are working for muscle gain. Where most people can simply rely on vegetables, fruits, grains, etc., to meet their energy needs, athletes should look into the diet very carefully and manage the high-protein to carb ratio while maintaining the intake of micronutrients and trace minerals. In a nutshell, a vegan bodybuilding diet is entirely different from a basic plant-based diet, as it is targeted to meet the need of building muscles.

Potential Benefits of the Vegan Bodybuilding Diet

Besides high-protein plant-based alternatives, this diet can provide several other health benefits to a bodybuilder. Let see how this diet can beat the negative effects of a non-vegan dietary approach and how well it can turn out to be for all those who are struggling to gain physical fitness.

1. **Reduces heart disease risk**

People consuming animal meat and fats are at more risk of developing heart diseases. The problem basically starts with bad cholesterol, also known as low-density lipoproteins. LDL is largely present in animal or saturated fats and it has the tendency to deposit into the blood vessels. The LDL is present in some amount in all the animal products from meat to dairy. A diet rich in those products can increase the LDL intake which consequently causes heart problems due to obstruction of blood vessels.

The vegan diet provides alternative cholesterol known as high-density lipoproteins, the good cholesterol which can bind the LDL with itself and removes it out of the blood. It does not deposit into the blood vessels and prevents several heart diseases.

2. **Can promote a healthy body weight**

For bodybuilders and athletes, there is a constant strive for an ideal or healthy body weight. When the vegan diet is compared to any traditional diet, the results clearly show how well it helps in maintaining body mass index. The plant-based diet does not add up to the body fats. For zero-fat body weight, the vegan diet seems idea for the physical fitness of every person involved in athletic activities. Since it can maintain body weight, it also keeps the problems of insulin resistance and low metabolic activities away from the person.

3. **Protects against certain cancers**

Nearly everyone vulnerable to cancer, or the ones suffering from the early stages of it, are prescribed the plant-based diet. There are many features of this diet that can prevent or treat the negative effects of cancer. Firstly, the plants with their phytonutrients have a therapeutic tendency and heal the cellular mutation that can cause cancer. Moreover, this diet makes the body resistant and strong towards the deleterious effects of cancer.

The Plant-Based Athlete

Dr. David C Nieman, the director of the Human Performance Laboratory at Appalachia State University in North Carolina, has studied the effects of diet on athletes and their fitness. His subject of study focused on physical fitness and its association with a plant-based or vegan diet.

Dr. Nieman is himself a marathon runner and happens to be a vegetarian. It was his personal interest to learn more about the effects of a vegan diet. According to him, the vegan diet can only prove healthy for the people who are involved in extreme physical exercises and remain engaged in such activities for more than an hour. He suggests a high-protein, low-carb vegan diet to control carb intake. In this way, a person can gain more muscle endurance and improvement in overall body shape and size.

There are also other studies that correlate the vegan diet and physical performance of a person. However, the work in this area is limited so far. However, there are many examples to look up to for inspiration. There are plenty of bodybuilders out there who are vegan and still manage to maintain an ideal body mass index, excellent muscle shape, and a great size.

Torre Washington is a good example. He has practically never tasted meat in his life but no one can guess that with the looks of his muscles and body shape. He was raised in a vegetarian family and grew up eating all kinds of plant-based food. Today he is a certified coach at the National Academy of Sports Medicine and a professional bodybuilder and a sprinter. He switched to veganism about twenty years ago, and he has become a vegan bodybuilding champion though his tailored vegan diet. Torre is a living example of how a vegan diet can best support muscle growth.

Nimai Delgado is another example that comes to mind when we discuss veganism and bodybuilding. Nimai has won the Fresno classic USA championships, Sacramento Pro, Hawaii Pro, and Grand Prix due to his well-maintained physique. He is now a professional bodybuilder and athlete. He was also a vegetarian from early childhood, and later switched to a 95% vegan diet back in 2015. His muscle shape and size are good enough to give a befitting response to all the critics of the vegan bodybuilding diet.

Patrik Baboumian, an Armenian-German athlete, has also proved the power of plant protein through his great shape and rock-solid muscles. Patrik has been using a vegan diet for the last five years of his twenty-three-year career. And today he feels stronger than ever before. He is quite vocal about the benefits of a vegan diet for bodybuilding and he also uses his social media accounts to debunk all the myths around veganism.

Protein and Recovery

Muscle fatigue, exhaustion, and pain are all the common symptoms of heavy workouts and physical training. Every time a person is involved in strenuous exercises, the muscles go through some degradation. Such muscles can regain their strength with better recovery and a good protein source. It is not the mere calories or carbohydrates that provide strength to the muscles, but the proteins. Energy is like fuel to a machine but without the basic building blocks, no machine can work effectively even in the abundance of that fuel. That means if a muscle is worn out, it requires more protein for its recovery.

There is no question about the importance of protein in muscle building; the focus of concern is how much protein is sufficient to support muscle recovery. The type and timing of protein is also important in this regard.

How Much Protein is Needed?

Dietary reference intake (DRI) is the standard index that indicates the number of nutrients that should be consumed at any age. The DRI protein for people older than 18 years is 0.8 grams of protein per kilogram of body weight in a day.

However, bodybuilders and athletes require more protein per kilograms of body weight to speed up their muscle recovery. The American Dietetic Association (ADA), Dieticians of Canada (DC), and the American College of Sports Medicine (ACSM) all support this argument of high protein requirement for muscle recovery.

The experts are of the view that protein is needed to recover the muscles and help in adaptation in different ways. For example, it can help in repairing the muscle fibers that are damaged during the exercises. It also transforms and strengthens the muscle fibers in order to make it adaptable to new lifestyle changes and exercises through protein synthesis, and aids in the replenishment process of the depleted energy reserves.

For high muscle endurance, the ACSM, ADA, and DC all recommend 1.2–1.4 grams of protein per kilogram of body weight in a day. However, if an athlete is engaged in resistance exercises, then the value should be as high as 1.7 grams of protein per kilogram of body weight in a day. This protein requirement can be met by a mere diet and some extra supplements if needed.

Protein Muscle Synthesis

It is a known fact that protein is a major building block of our muscles. Protein is a structural element and only plays its part in building and repairing the existing body cells. As our muscles grow and work, they constantly use protein. For a muscle to grow, proteins are an essential process, which allows new proteins to be produced. Muscle protein synthesis is closely linked with the muscles, much like a wall with bricks. To raise the wall to a new height or width, we need to add more bricks. Similarly, proteins are required to repair and grow the muscles.

There are two processes that are simultaneously occurring within our muscles and even in our bodies: the destructive and constructive processes. As the muscles become exhausted through physical activity, they will shed the used proteins through muscle protein breakdown, also known as proteolysis. This muscle degradation is important for protein synthesis; it acts as a trigger for the body to use more proteins for muscle building. That is why the more a person uses his muscles, the more proteins will be exhausted, and it will call for protein synthesis.

This protein synthesis cannot be carried out on its own. We need to provide the body with enough resources to synthesize muscle proteins. In order to grow the muscles in size, the process of protein synthesis must exceed the proteolysis or muscle breakdown. A high-protein diet is a source of the excess protein which can lead to better protein synthesis and muscle growth. The net protein balance of our muscles is equal to the difference between muscle protein synthesis and protein breakdown. A diet rich in proteins can ensure a higher net protein balance of the muscles. Nutrition plays a vital role in muscle growth and protein building.

Chapter 2: Macros and Micros

A good diet is all about the balance between the macro and micronutrients. While most people focus on the macros intake and stuck between carbs, proteins, and fats, they overlook the importance of the micronutrients that are equally essential in carrying out major metabolic activities in the body. In this section, we shall see how bodybuilders can maintain their daily nutritional intake and what are sources of those nutrients in the vegan diet. Before getting into the details of the micro and macronutrients, let us first see what are plant-based protein sources of a bodybuilder.

Plant-Based Protein Sources

The following are the known sources of proteins, and they should be added to a vegan diet to make it rich in proteins.

- **Beans and legumes:** These are an excellent source of protein. There are lots of fibers present in legumes and beans. However, they are also rich in carbs, so their intake should be limited in a day or per serving.
- **Hemp, flax, sunflower, and chia seeds:** Seeds are a great source of protein and omega 3s. Where vegans can't have seafood and meat, they can meet their protein needs with plant-based seeds. They are also full of essential oils.
- **Quinoa and amaranth:** They are also known as the pseudo-grains because they are low-carb grains and serve as the best option for bodybuilders. They are full of proteins and make up a healthy breakfast.
- **Meat substitutes:** There are several peas and soy-based products which can be used as a substitute for meat like tempeh, or tofu, etc. Edamame, soy protein powder, and soymilk are other good sources of protein.
- **Plant-based milk and yogurts:** Coconut milk, coconut cream, yogurt, etc.
- **Spirulina:** A blue-green algae which is full of proteins, vitamins, and minerals. It is great to add to smoothies and shakes.
- There are several **vegan protein powders** that can be used in snacks, desserts, and energy bars.
- **Nutritional yeast:** It is most often used in doughs and baked goods; the yeast is mixed with vitamin B12 during production, and it is also a good source of protein.
- **Sprouted grain bread:** These breads not only provide us with protein, but they are also a good source of complex carbohydrates.
- **Oats:** Often used in oatmeal, the oats are rich in protein, and they are full of fibers. Overnight oatmeal and oats porridges with fruits are a good option for a vegan diet.
- **Fruit and vegetables:** Though not all vegetables and fruits contain high doses of protein, they sure complement the vegan diet well by providing lots of fiber and calories.
- **Whole grains and cereals:** All grains and cereal are proven to be a good source of fibers, vitamin B, and protein.

- **Nuts and nut butter:** Nuts are good for a vegan diet due to their rich protein content, and nut butter is a perfect substitute for animal-based butter or fats. Peanut butter and almond butter can be used in this regard.
- **Tahini:** It is a thick paste made out of sesame seeds, and like its source, it is also full of protein and essential oils.
- **Healthy oils:** All plant-based oil is considered healthy for a vegan diet. There are some plant oils that are rich in omega 3s like avocado oil, hempseeds, and olive oil.
- **Vegan dark chocolate:** Dark chocolate is a good source of antioxidants and has all the necessary micronutrients which are essential for a vegan diet like vitamins A, B, E, magnesium, iron, potassium, and calcium.

Food to Avoid on a Plant-Based Diet

Where we have discussed the vegan sources of proteins and the food that is suitable for this diet, it is important to have a quick overview of the things that should be avoided:

- Eggs, dairy, meat, fish, poultry, and products produced by bees are strictly restricted on the plant-based diet. Similarly, food that contains any part of those items or that are extracted from them is also forbidden. Animal-based preservatives should also be avoided.
- There are some other ingredients that may be vegan in composition but for a vegan diet that is used for physical fitness, items like deep-fried foods, fast foods, candy, fried chips, etc., should be avoided.
- Junk food, whether it is vegan or not, is always unhealthy and should be looked out for. Things like ice cream or protein bars that say they are vegan should still be avoided because of the high dose of refined carbs they carry.

Macronutrients

Macronutrients are responsible for providing energy and basic building blocks to the body. Lack of these nutrients directly causes malnutrition and all the related health problems. They are required in large amounts for body growth and daily functioning. The sources of macronutrients in a plant-based diet are as follows:

1. **Protein sources**

Protein is most important to look for on a plant-based bodybuilding diet. You can find a good amount of protein in the following food items:

- Tempeh
- Tofu
- Seitan
- Edamame
- Lentils
- Chickpeas
- Nutritional yeast
- Quinoa
- Hempseed
- Peas
- Amaranth
- Tiff
- Oats

2. **Carb sources**

Carbohydrates are essential for metabolic activities, but their intake should be controlled to avoid a glucose spike in the blood and to prevent insulin resistance. Complex carbohydrates are considered healthier than refined carbs like those

present in sugar. On a plant-based vegan diet, the following are good options for carb intake:
- Black/brown rice
- Sweet potatoes
- Quinoa
- Lentils
- Oats
- Limited amount of bread and pasta.

3. Fat sources

Plants are an excellent source of healthy unsaturated fats, and you can use them from the following sources for a vegan diet:
- Avocado
- Flax seeds
- Chia seeds
- Almonds
- Almond butter
- Brazil nuts
- Walnuts
- Pumpkin seeds
- Cashew nuts
- Coconut

Micronutrient Intake

Nutrients that are required in small and trace amounts by the body but yet are vital for metabolic activities. They are the catalyst to many of the enzymic cavities and their deficiency can lead to serious health problems. Being on a vegan diet does restrict a person from getting a healthy number of micronutrients; there are many plant-based options for these nutrients, as follows:

1. Vitamin B12

Vitamin B12 is largely found in plants that are grown in a B12-rich soil. Organic products like mushrooms, nutritional yeast, noir, and spirulina are all full of B12. The deficiency of B12 can hamper the normal production of red blood cells. This can deprive the muscles of much-needed energy and oxygen. Most of the soil-grown vegetables lose their B12 when washed or cooked. The best way to maintain the healthy intake of B12 is to use products that are fortified with B12 such as plant milk, cereals, soy products, and yeast.

2. Vitamin D

This fat-soluble vitamin plays a major role in the absorption of calcium and phosphorus. Vitamin D deficiency can also lead to bone weakness despite normal calcium intake. A small amount of vitamin D is present in plant-based food but mostly can be sourced directly from the sunlight. People who don't go out much in the sunlight suffer from its deficiency. Sitting for just 15 minutes in the sun is important to absorb vitamin D.

3. Long-chain omega-3s

Omega fatty acids are largely present in seafood, so it is assumed that a plant-based diet can deprive us of the much-needed omega 3 and omega 6, but that is not true. There are certain algae oils, sunflower seeds, hemp seeds, and other seeds that are rich in omega 3 fatty acids—whereas the need for omega 6 fatty acids can be met with the use of sunflower oil, sesame oils, safflower, and corn oils.

4. Iodine

For a normal thyroid function, iodine is essential to consume. The thyroid is responsible for controlling our metabolic rate, and the inefficiency of the thyroid leads to poor metabolic activity. Iodine is not largely present in the food we eat, but it is added to salt to produce iodized salt. This salt can maintain the level of iodine in the blood.

5. Iron

Iron is vital to red blood cells and to the formation of new DNA. It is capable of carrying oxygen and aids in energy metabolism. Its deficiency can, therefore, lead to several health problems. Vegans should focus on their iron intake and look for the ingredients which are rich in iron like seeds, nuts, dry fruits, beans, vegetables, and peas. There are special iron-fortified products in the market like iron-fortified bread, cereals, plant milk, etc., which should be added to the diet.

6. Calcium

Calcium is the mineral that supports bone growth and repair which is important to sustain muscle growth, especially when a person is weight lifting. It is also essential for muscle function, cardiac function, and nerve impulse. Lack of calcium can sometimes cause muscle stiffness, spasms, or weakness. Plant-based food that is rich in calcium mainly includes turnip greens, watercress, chickpeas, broccoli, calcium tofu, kale, bok choy, and calcium-fortified juice and milk.

The average calcium intake should not be less than 525 mg per day. Calcium supplements can also be used to meet an individual's needs.

7. Zinc

Zinc is another mineral that is vital for better immunity, metabolism, and cell repair. Vegans can maximize their zinc intake by consuming more whole grains, seeds, nuts, legumes, tofu, and wheat germ. Fermented foods such as miso, sauerkraut, and tempeh are also good for zinc intake. Soak legumes, seeds, and nuts in water overnight and then eat them to increase the absorption of zinc in the body.

Chapter 3: Plant-Based Supplements

Bodybuilding is extreme and drains the body faster than any other physical activity. A simple diet can provide much-needed energy and nutrients but it is not enough to maximize the muscle potential that is required for bodybuilding and athletics. Therefore, special supplements are needed to boost muscle growth. Since most of the protein supplements commonly available in the market are animal-sourced, they should be avoided. However, there are specific options for vegans:

1. Protein powder

Protein powder is extracted from plant-based sources and is an easier way to meet all protein needs as well as maintain net muscle protein balance. Protein powder can be mixed in smoothies, baked goods, and desserts. The commonly recommended plant-based protein powders include:

- Sunwarrior protein powder
- Vega protein powder
- Garden of Life
- PlantFusion

These supplements should be used with care, in an adequate amount.

2. BCAAs

Branch Chain Amino Acids, or BCAAs, are the types of amino acids that our body cannot produce on its own, so it needs to be consumed from external sources. Although BCAAs are also present in most of the plant-based proteins, it is always good to have some backup source for the hard training days. It can be consumed before or after the exercises and the workout sessions. They help in quick and improved recovery of the muscles after the exercise and help maintain the glycogen reserves. Buy yourself supplements which have a higher leucine to valine and isoleucine ratio (amino acids).

3. Creatine

Studies have shown that muscle strength and mass can be maximized by creatine. Creatine is largely found in animal-based sources. However, it is also producing by the human liver in some amount. Vegans have therefore comparatively lower levels of creatine in their blood. This level can be enhanced by supporting the liver function with a healthy diet and by taking supplements like Optimal Nutrition.

4. NAC

NAC, or N-acetylcysteine, is a cysteine amino acid, and it is a comparatively stable form of protein that is easily absorbed in the body. NAC is discovered as that miraculous amino acid which can increase physical performance and reduces the oxidative stress of the cells. It is responsible for increasing levels of glutathione in the body.

5. Ashwagandha

Indian ginseng, or ashwagandha, is full of healing benefits. Its tea is famous in traditional Indian cuisine due to the obvious advantages. This herb has also been used as medicine in most parts of the world. If you are looking for a natural supplement to boost your muscle recovery, then do add ashwagandha powder to your smoothies every now and then.

This herb has the ability to boost the production of testosterone in males by 15%, which helps to greatly increase in muscle strength and mass. It is both available in powder and pill forms.

This supplement can also reduce anxiety and stress due to the cortisol and c-reactive proteins. Superfoods Organic Ashwagandha root powder is recommended.

Cheat Days

It is important to give yourself a break from a diet in order to gain consistency. Most people give up on a diet because they become too hard on themselves. Cheat days are a way to keep yourself on track and curb your cravings. However, there are certain cheat day mistakes that cost too much for a bodybuilder who has worked hard to get his body in shape. Those common mistakes are:
1. Frequent Cheating
2. Excessive eating on the cheating days
3. Too much dietary fat intake
4. Drinking too much alcohol and sugary beverages

Even on your cheat days, keep your vegan lifestyle in mind and remind yourself of the caloric needs of the body. Cheating frequently and eating too much unhealthy food can get you off track, and can cause greater weight gain than usual. During your cheat days you can have things like:
1. Vegan ice creams
2. Protein bars
3. Cauliflower-crusted pizza
4. Vegan cookies

Management and Fitness Goals

Muscle growth and maintenance is all about management. Set your fitness goals and then follow the diet to meet those specific targets. Divide your goals into small achievable targets and then see the results. Here are some important points to keep in mind:

1. Self-discipline

It all starts with self-discipline; without you taming your mind, you cannot tame your body into a desired size and shape. The vegan bodybuilder must realize that this diet is as beneficial as any other animal-based diet. We just need to focus on the nutritional intake and must learn to maintain the proportion of the ingredients to meet the protein and caloric needs of the body.

2. Frequent and small meals

An effective strategy to keep the body fat free, maintain body weight, and increase muscle mass is to reduce the size of the meal and increase the frequency of daily meals. Each meal should carry more proteins than carbs and fats. It should also have a mix of all the essential micronutrients. With small and frequents meals, you constantly provide energy to the muscles to repair and rebuild while keeping the overall body weight maintained.

3. Grams per body weight

In the vegan bodybuilding diet, the important thing is to consider the proportion of nutrients in comparison to body weight. Perhaps, in this diet, there is no one-size-fits-all formula. Rather, every bodybuilder must consume proteins and other macronutrients as per the body's needs and weight. Consume proteins according to your body weight and size to maximize muscle growth.

4. Calories

During strenuous exercises, our muscles burn a large number of calories to gain energy, which creates a constant demand for energy. Even when the muscles repair themselves, they need the energy to do so. Therefore, it is important to keep the caloric intake in check. Excessive calories are also not suitable for bodybuilders as it may lead to weight gain; the balance should be maintained.

5. 30% fat only

The total fat intake should only constitute 30% of the meal. This percentage is a standard limit for all. A higher fat intake would lead to the deposition of fats in the body and leads to obesity; 30% fat is enough to meet the basic fat needs of a body and prevents weight gain and other related problems.

6. Consistent efforts

Just exercise and physical activities cannot guarantee good health and strong muscles—that has to be supported by a consistent effort and good diet. A person on a weight control diet has to be more cautious of his food preferences, portion size, and the bodily consumption of that food. Without consistency, all efforts are vain.

ESSENTIAL RECIPES

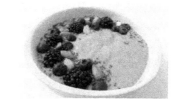

Green Smoothie Bowl

Preparation time: 10 minutes
Total time: 10 minutes
Servings: 2

Ingredients
Smoothie Bowl
- 2 cups fresh spinach
- 1 medium avocado, peeled, pitted, and chopped roughly
- 2 scoops unsweetened vegan protein powder
- 3 tablespoons maple syrup
- 2 tablespoons fresh lemon juice
- 1 cup unsweetened almond milk
- ¼ cup ice cubes

Topping
- 2 tablespoons chia seeds
- 2 tablespoons fresh blueberries
- 2 tablespoons fresh blackberries
- 1 tablespoon almonds
- 1 tablespoon pistachios

How to Prepare
1. In a high-speed blender, add all the ingredients and pulse until smooth.
2. Transfer into 2 serving bowls and serve with topping ingredients.

Nutritional Values
- Calories 464
- Total Fat 24.6 g
- Saturated Fat 4.2 g
- Cholesterol 0 mg
- Sodium 993 mg
- Total Carbs 36.2 g
- Fiber 10.7 g
- Sugar 20.2 g
- Protein 31.2 g

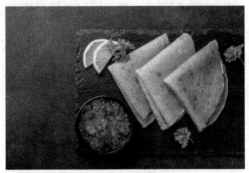

Savory Crepes

Preparation time: 10 minutes
Cooking time: 20 minutes
Total time: 30 minutes
Servings: 4

Ingredients
- 1¼ cups chickpea flour
- 1½ cups water
- ¼ teaspoon garlic powder
- ¼ teaspoon red chili powder
- Salt, as required

How to Prepare
1. In a blender, add all the ingredients and pulse until well combined.
2. Heat a lightly greased non-stick skillet over medium-high heat.
3. Add the desired amount of the mixture and tilt the pan to spread it evenly.
4. Cook for about 3 minutes.
5. Carefully, flip the crepe and cook for about 1-2 minutes.
6. Repeat with the remaining mixture.
7. Serve warm.

Nutritional Values
- Calories 229
- Total Fat 3.8 g
- Saturated Fat 0.4 g
- Cholesterol 0 mg
- Sodium 55 mg
- Total Carbs 38.1 g
- Fiber 11 g
- Sugar 6.7 g
- Protein 12.1 g

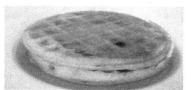

Blueberry Waffles

Preparation time: 10 minutes
Cooking time: 24 minutes
Total time: 34 minutes
Servings: 6

Ingredients
- 2 cups almond flour
- 2 cups oat flour
- 2 tablespoons cornstarch
- 2 tablespoons baking powder
- 1 teaspoon ground cinnamon
- ½ teaspoon salt
- 4 tablespoons maple syrup, plus extra for drizzling
- 3 cups unsweetened almond milk
- 1 teaspoon vanilla extract
- 1 cup fresh blueberries

How to Prepare
1. In a large bowl, mix together the flours, cornstarch, baking powder, cinnamon, and salt.
2. Add the almond milk and vanilla and mix until just combined.
3. Gently, fold in the blueberries.
4. Preheat the waffle iron and then grease it.
5. Place the desired amount of the mixture into the preheated waffle iron and cook for about 5–6 minutes or until golden-brown.
6. Repeat with the remaining mixture.
7. Serve warm with the drizzling of extra maple syrup.

Nutritional Values
- Calories 431
- Total Fat 21.6 g
- Saturated Fat 2 g
- Cholesterol 0 mg
- Sodium 303 mg
- Total Carbs 47.6 g
- Fiber 8.4 g
- Sugar 10.4 g
- Protein 12.7 g

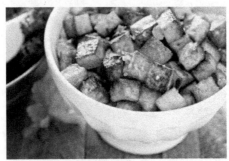

Baked Tofu

Preparation time: 15 minutes
Cooking time: 30 minutes
Total time: 45 minutes
Servings: 3

Ingredients
- 1 (14-ounce) package extra-firm tofu, drained, pressed, and cubed
- 1 tablespoon cornstarch
- 1 tablespoon low-sodium soy sauce
- 1 tablespoon olive oil
- Freshly ground black pepper, to taste

How to Prepare
1. Preheat the oven to 400ºF and line a large, rimmed baking sheet with parchment paper.
2. In a bowl, add all the ingredients and toss to coat well.
3. Arrange the tofu cubes onto the prepared baking sheet in a single layer.
4. Bake for about 25–30 minutes, tossing once halfway through.
5. Serve hot.

Nutritional Values
- Calories 172
- Total Fat 12.4 g
- Saturated Fat 1.4 g
- Cholesterol 0 mg
- Sodium 304 mg
- Total Carbs 5.4.1 g
- Fiber 0.6 g
- Sugar 1 g
- Protein 13.4 g

Chickpeas Falafel Bowl

Preparation time: 25 minutes
Cooking time: 30 minutes
Total time: 55 minutes
Servings: 4

Ingredients

Falafels
- 1 cupdried chickpeas, rinsed, picked over, and soaked for12–24 hours in the refrigerator
- ½ cupred onion, chopped roughly
- 4garlic cloves, peeled
- ½ cupfresh cilantro
- ½ cup fresh parsley
- 1 tablespoon olive oil
- ½ teaspoonground cumin
- Salt and ground black pepper, to taste

Dressing
- ¼ cup tahini
- 2 garlic cloves, minced
- 2 tablespoons fresh lemon juice
- 1 tablespoon white miso
- ¼ cup water

Salad
- 3 large tomatoes, sliced
- 4 cups lettuce, torn

How to Prepare

1. Preheat the oven to 375ºF. Place a rack in the middle of the oven. Generously, grease a large rimmed baking sheet.
2. For falafel: in a food processor, add all the ingredients and pulse until smooth.
3. Take about 2 tablespoons of the mixture and shape it into a ½-inch thick patty.
4. Repeat with the remaining mixture.
5. Arrange the patties onto the prepared baking sheet in a single layer.
6. Bake for about 25–30 minutes, flipping once halfway through.
7. Meanwhile, for dressing: in a bowl, add all the ingredients and beat until well combined.
8. Divide salad ingredients and falafel patties into serving bowls evenly.
9. Drizzle with dressing and serve immediately.

Nutritional Values

- Calories 360
- Total Fat 15.4 g
- Saturated Fat 2.1 g
- Cholesterol 0 mg
- Sodium 246 mg
- Total Carbs 45.3 g
- Fiber 13.1 g
- Sugar 10.7 g
- Protein 15 g

Glazed Carrots

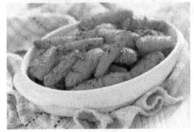

Preparation time: 10 minutes
Cooking time: 15 minutes
Total time: 25 minutes
Servings: 4

Ingredients
- 2 cups of water
- 1 pound baby carrots
- 3 tablespoons maple syrup
- 1 tablespoon coconut oil
- Salt, to taste
- 1 tablespoon fresh lemon juice
- 2 tablespoons fresh parsley, chopped
- Ground black pepper, to taste
- 1 tablespoon fresh parsley, minced

How to Prepare
1. In a medium pan, add the water over medium-high heat and bring to a boil.
2. Add the carrots and again bring to a boil.
3. Reduce the heat to medium and cook for about 6–8 minutes.
4. Drain the carrots well.
5. In a skillet, add the maple syrup, coconut oil, lemon juice, salt, and black pepper and cook for about 5 minutes, stirring continuously.
6. Stir in the parsley and remove from the heat.

Nutritional Values
- Calories 110
- Total Fat 3.6 g
- Saturated Fat 3 g
- Cholesterol 0 mg
- Sodium 131 mg
- Total Carbs 19.7 g
- Fiber 3.4 g
- Sugar 14.4 g
- Protein 0.98 g

Barley & Chickpea Soup

Preparation time: 15 minutes
Cooking time: 1½ hours
Total time: 1¾ hours
Servings: 8

Ingredients
- 1 cup pearl barley
- 1 (15-ounce) can chickpeas, rinsed and drained
- 2 large carrots, peeled and chopped
- 1 zucchini, chopped
- 2 celery stalks, chopped
- 1 red onion, chopped
- 2 cups tomatoes, chopped
- 1 teaspoon dried parsley, crushed
- 1 teaspoon curry powder
- 1 teaspoon paprika
- 3 bay leaves
- Salt and ground black pepper, to taste
- 5 cups homemade vegetable broth
- 4 cups water
- ½ cup fresh cilantro, chopped

How to Prepare
1. In a large soup pan, add all the ingredients (except parsley) over high heat and bring to a boil.
2. Lower the heat to medium-low and simmer, covered for about 1½ hours.
3. Remove from the heat and discard the bay leaves.
4. Serve hot with the garnishing of cilantro.

Nutritional Values
- Calories 326
- Total Fat 4.8 g
- Saturated Fat 0.7 g
- Cholesterol 0 mg
- Sodium 537 mg
- Total Carbs 55.8 g
- Fiber 15.1 g
- Sugar 9.5 g
- Protein 17.3 g

Lentil Soup

Preparation time: 15 minutes
Cooking time: 35 minutes
Total time: 50 minutes
Servings: 4

Ingredients
- 1 tablespoon vegetable oil
- 1 cup yellow onion, chopped
- ½ cup carrots, peeled and chopped
- ½ cup celery, chopped
- 2 garlic cloves, minced
- 4 cups vegetable broth
- 2½ cups sweet potatoes, peeled and chopped
- 1 cup red lentils, rinsed
- 1½ tablespoons fresh lemon juice
- Salt and ground black pepper, to taste
- 2 tablespoons fresh cilantro, chopped

How to Prepare
1. In a large Dutch oven, heat the oil over medium heat and sauté the onion, carrots, and celery for about 5–7 minutes.
2. Add the garlic and sauté for about 1 minute.
3. Add the sweet potatoes and cook for about 1–2 minutes.
4. Add in the broth and bring to a boil.
5. Lower the heat to low and simmer, covered for about 5 minutes.
6. Stir in the red lentils and again bring to a boil over medium-high heat.
7. Lower the heat to low and simmer, covered for about 15–20 minutes, or until desired doneness.
8. Add the lemon juice, salt, and black pepper, and remove from the heat.
9. Serve hot with the garnishing of cilantro.

Nutritional Values
- Calories 471
- Total Fat 5.6 g
- Saturated Fat 1.2 g
- Cholesterol 0 mg
- Sodium 836 mg
- Total Carbs 61 g
- Fiber 19.7 g
- Sugar 4.4 g
- Protein 19.3 g

Beans & Pasta Stew

Preparation time: 15 minutes
Cooking time: 35 minutes
Total time: 50 minutes
Servings: 6

Ingredients
- ¼ cup canola oil
- 1 large yellow onion, chopped
- 1 potato, chopped
- 8 ounces fresh shiitake mushrooms, sliced
- 1 medium tomato, chopped
- 2 tablespoons garlic, chopped finely
- 2 bay leaves
- 2 tablespoons mixed Italian herbs (rosemary, thyme, basil), chopped
- 1 teaspoon cayenne pepper
- 4 cups homemade vegetable broth
- 2 tablespoons apple cider vinegar
- 1/3 cup nutritional yeast
- 1/3 cup roasted tomato salsa
- 8 ounces fresh collard greens
- 1 cup whole-wheat fusilli pasta
- 1 (15-ounce) can cannellini beans, drained and rinsed
- Salt and ground black pepper, to taste

How to Prepare
1. In a large pan, heat the oil over medium heat and sauté the onion, mushrooms, potato, and tomato for about 4–5 minutes.
2. Add the garlic, bay leaves, herbs, and cayenne pepper and sauté for about 1 minute.
3. Add the broth and bring to a boil.
4. Stir in the vinegar, pasta, nutritional yeast, and tomato salsa and again bring to a boil.
5. Lower the heat to medium-low and simmer, covered for about 20 minutes.
6. Uncover and stir in the greens and beans.
7. Simmer for about 4–5 minutes.
8. Stir in the salt and black pepper and remove from the heat.
9. Serve hot.

Nutritional Values
- Calories 299
- Total Fat 11.3 g
- Saturated Fat 1 g
- Cholesterol 0 mg
- Sodium 701 mg
- Total Carbs 37.2 g
- Fiber 12.3 g
- Sugar 4 g
- Protein 16 g

Mocha Tofu Pudding

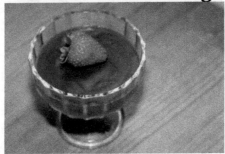

Preparation time: 15 minutes
Total time: 15 minutes
Servings: 4

Ingredients
- 16 ounces silken tofu, pressed and drained
- 1/3 cup cacao powder
- 1 tablespoon instant coffee
- 2 teaspoons vanilla extract
- ¼ cup maple syrup
- ¼ cup fresh strawberries

How to Prepare
1. In a blender, add all ingredients (except the raspberries) and pulse until creamy and smooth.
2. Transfer into serving bowls and refrigerate to chill for at least 2 hours.
3. Garnish with raspberries and serve.

Nutritional Values
- Calories 147
- Total Fat 4.5 g
- Saturated Fat 1.3 g
- Cholesterol 0 mg
- Sodium 43 mg
- Total Carbs 20.2 g
- Fiber 2.3 g
- Sugar 13.9 g
- Protein 9.2 g

BREAKFAST RECIPES

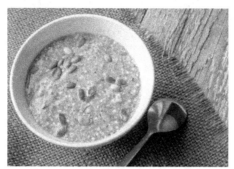

Overnight Porridge

Preparation time: 10 minutes
Total time: 10 minutes
Servings: 2

Ingredients
- 2/3 cup plus ¼ cup unsweetened coconut milk, divided
- ½ cup hemp hearts
- 1 tablespoon chia seed
- 3–4 drops liquid stevia
- ½ teaspoon vanilla extract
- Pinch of salt
- 2 tablespoons pumpkin seeds

How to Prepare
1. In a larger airtight container, place 2/3 cup of the coconut milk, hemp hearts, chia seed, stevia, vanilla extract, and salt, and stir until well combined.
2. Cover the container tightly and refrigerate overnight.
3. Just before serving, add the remaining coconut milk and stir to combine.
4. Serve immediately.

Nutritional Values
- Calories 460
- Total Fat 38 g
- Saturated Fat 16.9 g
- Cholesterol 0 mg
- Sodium 114 mg
- Total Carbs 10 g
- Fiber 5.6 g
- Sugar 3 g
- Protein 17.6 g

Pumpkin Porridge

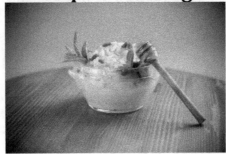

Preparation time: 15 minutes
Cooking time: 25 minutes
Total time: 40 minutes
Servings: 4

Ingredients
- 1 cup water
- Pinch of salt
- 1 cup almond flour
- 2 tablespoons maple syrup
- ½ cup sugar-free pumpkin puree
- ½ teaspoon ground cinnamon
- Pinch of ground nutmeg
- ½ cup almonds, chopped

How to Prepare
1. In a pan, add the water and salt over medium-high heat and bring to a boil.
2. Slowly, add the almond flour, stirring continuously.
3. Lower the heat to medium and cook for about 15–20 minutes, or until all the liquid is absorbed, stirring continuously.
4. Add the remaining ingredients (except the almonds) and stir to combine well.
5. Remove the pan from the heat and serve immediately with the topping of almonds.

Nutritional Values
- Calories 274
- Total Fat 19.4 g
- Saturated Fat 1.5 g
- Cholesterol 0 mg
- Sodium 51 mg
- Total Carbs 18 g
- Fiber 5.5 g
- Sugar 7.5 g
- Protein 9 g

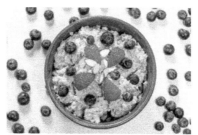

Quinoa, Oats, & Seeds Porridge

Preparation time: 10 minutes
Cooking time: 15 minutes
Total time: 25 minutes
Servings: 3

Ingredients
- 2 cups unsweetened almond milk
- 2 cups water
- 1 cup old-fashioned oats
- ¼ cup dried quinoa, rinsed
- 1 tablespoon flax seeds
- 1 tablespoon chia seeds
- 3 tablespoons maple syrup
- ½ teaspoon vanilla extract
- 3 tablespoons almonds, chopped
- ¼ cup fresh strawberries, hulled and sliced
- ¼ cup fresh blueberries

How to Prepare
1. In a pan, mix together all the ingredients (except the pumpkin seeds and berries) over medium heat and bring to a gentle boil.
2. Cook for about 20 minutes, stirring occasionally.
3. Stir in chopped dates and immediately remove from heat.
4. Serve warm with the garnishing of berries and almonds.

Nutritional Values
- Calories 304
- Total Fat 9.6 g
- Saturated Fat 1 g
- Cholesterol 0 mg
- Sodium 130 mg
- Total Carbs 48 g
- Fiber 7.1 g
- Sugar 14.3 g
- Protein 8.9 g

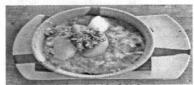

Barley Porridge

Preparation time: 10 minutes
Cooking time: 50 minutes
Total time: 1 hour
Servings: 3

Ingredients
- 3 cups water
- 1 cup pearl barley
- ¼ cup walnuts
- 2 tablespoons raisins
- 1 tablespoon maple syrup
- 1 teaspoon ground cinnamon
- ¼ teaspoon ground nutmeg
- 1 cup unsweetened soymilk
- 2 tablespoons pumpkin seeds
- 1 apple, cored and chopped

How to Prepare
1. In a pan, add the water over high heat and bring to a boil.
2. Add the barley and again bring to a boil.
3. Lower the heat to low and simmer, covered for about 35–40 minutes, or until most of liquid is absorbed.
4. Add the walnuts, raisins, maple syrup, cinnamon, and nutmeg and stir to combine.
5. Stir in ½ cup of the soymilk and cook for about 2–3 minutes.
6. Stir in the remaining soymilk and remove from the heat.
7. Serve warm with the topping of apple pieces.

Nutritional Values
- Calories 451
- Total Fat 11.2 g
- Saturated Fat 0 g
- Cholesterol 51 mg
- Sodium 79.2 mg
- Total Carbs 14.3 g
- Fiber 2.6 g
- Sugar 19.3 g
- Protein 31.6 g

Banana Pancakes

Preparation time: 15 minutes
Cooking time: 12 minutes
Total time: 27 minutes
Servings: 3

Ingredients
- 2 tablespoons flaxseed meal
- 5 tablespoons water
- 1½ cups rolled oats
- ¼ cup unsweetened vegan protein powder
- 1 teaspoon baking powder
- ½ teaspoon baking soda
- ¼ teaspoon salt
- 1½ cups unsweetened almond milk
- 2 tablespoons coconut oil, melted
- 2 teaspoons vanilla extract

How to Prepare
1. In a large bowl, add the flaxseed meal and water and mix well.
2. Set aside for about 10 minutes.
3. In another large bowl, add the oats, protein powder, baking powder, baking soda, and salt, and mix well.
4. In the bowl of flaxseed meal, add the almond milk, coconut oil, and vanilla extract and beat until well combined.
5. Add the almond milk mixture into the flour mixture and beat until well combined.
6. Set aside for about 10–12 minutes.
7. Heat a lightly greased skillet over medium heat.
8. Add desired amount of mixture and with a spoon, spread into an even layer.
9. Cook about 1–2 minutes per side.
10. Repeat with the remaining mixture.
11. Serve warm.

Nutritional Values
- Calories 326
- Total Fat 16.3 g
- Saturated Fat 8.7 g
- Cholesterol 0 mg
- Sodium 782 mg
- Total Carbs 31.2 g
- Fiber 5.9 g
- Sugar 0.8 g
- Protein 15.2 g

Spinach & Tomato Omelet

Preparation time: 15 minutes
Cooking time: 10 minutes
Total time: 25 minutes
Servings: 2

Ingredients
- ¾ cup chickpeas flour
- ½ teaspoon cumin seeds
- Salt and ground black pepper, to taste
- ½ cup water
- 1½ cups fresh spinach, chopped finely
- ½ cup tomato, seeded and chopped finely
- 1 green chili, chopped finely
- 2 tablespoons vegetable oil

How to Prepare
1. In a bowl, add the chickpeas flour, cumin seeds, salt, and black pepper, and mix well.
2. Slowly, add the water and mix until a smooth mixture is formed.
3. Add the vegetables and green chili and stir to combine.
4. In a non-stick skillet, heat 1 tablespoon of the oil over medium heat.
5. Add about ½ cup of the mixture into the skillet and with the back of a spoon, spread into a 7-inch circle.
6. Spread about 2 teaspoons of oil over the veggie mixture and cook for about 30 seconds.
7. Flip the omelet and cook for about 2–3 minutes, flipping and pressing the omelet 2–3 times.
8. Repeat with the remaining veggie mixture.
9. Serve hot.

Nutritional Values
- Calories 270
- Total Fat 16.2 g
- Saturated Fat 2.9 g
- Cholesterol 0 mg
- Sodium 123 mg
- Total Carbs 23 g
- Fiber 4.9 g
- Sugar 5.1 g
- Protein 9 g

Veggie Omelet

Preparation time: 15 minutes **Total time:** 38 minutes
Cooking time: 23 minutes **Servings:** 2

Ingredients

- 8 ounces fresh asparagus, trimmed and cut into 1-inch pieces
- ¼ of red bell pepper, seeded and chopped roughly
- ¼ of green bell pepper, seeded and chopped roughly
- 1 tablespoon fresh chives, chopped
- ¾ cup water
- ½ cup superfine chickpea flour
- 1 tablespoon chia seeds
- 2 tablespoons nutritional yeast
- ½ teaspoon baking powder
- 1 teaspoon dried basil, crushed
- ¼ teaspoon ground turmeric
- ¼ teaspoon red pepper flakes, crushed
- Salt and ground black pepper, to taste
- 1 small tomato, chopped

How to Prepare

1. In a pan of the lightly salted boiling water, add the asparagus and cook for about 5–7 minutes or until crisp tender.
2. Drain the asparagus well and set aside.
3. Meanwhile, in a bowl, add the bell peppers, chives, and water, and mix.
4. In another bowl, add the remaining ingredients (except tomato) and mix well.
5. Add the water mixture into the bowl of flour mixture and mix until well combined.
6. Set aside for at least 10 minutes.
7. Lightly, grease a large non-stick skillet and heat over medium heat
8. Add ½ of the mixture and with the back of a spoon, smooth it.
9. Sprinkle half of the tomato over mixture evenly.
10. With a lid, cover the skillet tightly and cook for about 4 minutes.
11. Now, place half of the cooked asparagus over one side of omelet.
12. Carefully, fold the other half over asparagus to cover it.
13. Cover the skillet and cook for 3–4 minutes more.
14. Repeat with the remaining mixture.
15. Serve warm.

Nutritional Values

- Calories 276
- Total Fat 5.2 g
- Saturated Fat 0.6 g
- Cholesterol 0 mg
- Sodium 105 mg
- Total Carbs 45.8 g
- Fiber 16 g
- Sugar 10.2 g
- Protein 18.3 g

Veggie Quiche

Preparation time: 20 minutes
Cooking time: 1 hour
Total time: 1¼ hours
Servings: 4

Ingredients

- 1 cup water
- Pinch of salt
- 1/3 cup bulgur wheat
- ¾ tablespoon light sesame oil
- 1½ cups fresh cremini mushrooms, sliced
- 1 tablespoon low-sodium soy sauce
- 2 cups fresh broccoli, chopped
- 1 yellow onion, chopped
- 16 ounces firm tofu, pressed and cubed
- ¾ tablespoon white miso
- 1¼ tablespoons tahini

How to Prepare

1. Preheat oven to 350ºF. Lightly, grease a pie dish.
2. In a pan, add the water over medium heat and salt, bring to a boil.
3. Stir in the bulgur and again bring to a rolling boil.
4. Reduce the heat to low and simmer, covered for about 12–15 minutes, or until all the liquid is absorbed.
5. Remove from heat and set the pan aside to cool slightly.
6. Now, place the cooked bulgur into the pie dish evenly and with your fingers, press into the bottom.
7. Bake for about 12 minutes.
8. Remove from the oven and set aside to cool slightly.
9. Meanwhile, in a skillet, heat oil over medium heat.
10. Add the mushrooms, broccoli, and onion and cook for about 10 minutes, stirring occasionally.
11. Remove from the heat and transfer into a large bowl to cool slightly.
12. Meanwhile, in a food processor, add the remaining ingredients and pulse until smooth.
13. Transfer the tofu mixture into the bowl with veggie mixture and mix until well combined.
14. Place the veggie mixture over the baked crust evenly.
15. Bake for about 30 minutes or until top becomes golden-brown.
16. Remove from the oven and set the pie dish aside for at least 10 minutes.
17. With a sharp knife, cut into 4 equal-sized slices and serve.

Nutritional Values

- Calories 211
- Total Fat 10.4 g
- Saturated Fat 1.8 g
- Cholesterol 0 mg
- Sodium 418 mg
- Total Carbs 19.6 g
- Fiber 5.7 g
- Sugar 3.6 g
- Protein 14.4 g

Fruity Muffins

Preparation time: 15 minutes
Cooking time: 20 minutes
Total time: 35 minutes
Servings: 6

Ingredients
- ½ cup hot water
- ¼ cup flaxseed meal
- 1 banana, peeled and sliced
- 1 apple, peeled, cored, and chopped roughly
- 2 cups rolled oats
- ½ cup walnuts, chopped
- ½ cup raisins
- ¼ teaspoon baking soda
- 2 tablespoons ground cinnamon
- ½ cup unsweetened almond milk
- ¼ cup maple syrup

How to Prepare
1. Preheat the oven to 350ºF and line a 12-cup muffin tin with paper liners.
2. In a bowl, add water and flaxseed and beat until well combined. Set aside for about 5 minutes.
3. In a blender, add the flaxseed mixture and remaining ingredients and pulse until smooth and creamy.
4. Transfer the mixture into prepared muffin cups evenly.
5. Bake for about 20 minutes or until a toothpick inserted in the center comes out clean.
6. Remove the muffin tin from oven and place onto a wire rack to cool for about 10 minutes.
7. Carefully invert the muffins onto the wire rack to cool completely before serving.

Nutritional Values
- Calories 309
- Total Fat 9.9 g
- Saturated Fat 0.9 g
- Cholesterol 0 mg
- Sodium 73 mg
- Total Carbs 50.8 g
- Fiber 7.9 g
- Sugar 21.7 g
- Protein 8 g

Nuts, Seeds, & Coconut Granola

Preparation time: 15 minutes
Cooking time: 35 minutes
Total time: 50 minutes
Servings: 6

Ingredients

- ½ cup unsweetened coconut flakes
- 1 cup raw almonds
- 1 cup raw cashews
- ¼ cup raw sunflower seeds, shelled
- ¼ cup raw pumpkin seeds, shelled
- ¼ cup coconut oil
- ½ cup maple syrup
- 1 teaspoon vanilla extract
- ½ cup golden raisins
- ½ cup black raisins
- Salt, to taste

How to Prepare

1. Preheat the oven to 275°F. Line a large baking sheet with baking paper.
2. In a food processor, add the coconut flakes, almonds, cashews, and seeds, and pulse until chopped finely.
3. in a medium non-stick pan, add the oil, maple syrup, and vanilla on medium-high heat and cook for about 2–3 minutes, stirring continuously.
4. Remove from heat and immediately stir in nuts mixture.
5. Transfer the mixture onto the prepared baking sheet and spread evenly.
6. Bake for about 20–25 minutes, stirring twice.
7. Remove from oven and immediately stir in raisins.
8. Sprinkle with a little salt.
9. With the back of a spatula, flatten the surface of mixture.
10. Set aside to cool completely.
11. Then break the granola into desired size chunks.
12. Serve with your choice of non-dairy milk and fruit topping.

Nutritional Values

- Calories 546
- Total Fat 36.7 g
- Saturated Fat 15.8 g
- Cholesterol 0 mg
- Sodium 41 mg
- Total Carbs 51.1 g
- Fiber 5.3 g
- Sugar 32.6 g
- Protein 10.2 g

HIGH-PROTEIN SNACKS RECIPES
Spiced & Herbed Nuts

Preparation time: 10 minutes
Cooking time: 12 minutes
Total time: 22 minutes
Servings: 12

Ingredients
- 1½ cups whole almonds
- 1½ cups pistachios
- 1 cup pecan halves
- 1 cup walnut halves
- 1 cup cashews
- 1/3 cup extra-virgin olive oil
- 2 tablespoons fresh rosemary, chopped
- 2 tablespoons fresh thyme, chopped
- 2 tablespoons fresh oregano, chopped
- 1 tablespoon smoked paprika
- 1 teaspoon cayenne pepper
- 2 teaspoons garlic powder
- Salt, to taste

How to Prepare
1. Preheat your oven to 350ºF and line a large baking sheet with parchment paper.
2. In a bowl, place all ingredients and toss to coat well.
3. Transfer the nut mixture onto the prepared baking sheet and spread in a single layer.
4. Roast for about 10–12 minutes, flipping after every 5 minutes.
5. Remove from the oven and set the baking sheet aside to cool completely before serving.

Nutritional Values
- Calories 369
- Total Fat 34.3 g
- Saturated Fat 3.9 g
- Cholesterol 0 mg
- Sodium 55 mg
- Total Carbs 12 g
- Fiber 5.6 g
- Sugar 2.3 g
- Protein 10 g

Spicy Chickpeas

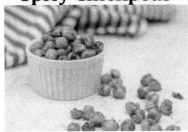

Preparation time: 10 minutes
Cooking time: 25 minutes
Total time: 35 minutes
Servings: 6

Ingredients
- 2 (15-ounce) cans chickpeas, rinsed and drained
- ¼ cup olive oil
- ½ teaspoon red chili powder
- ¾ teaspoon paprika
- ¾ teaspoon garlic powder
- ½ teaspoon onion powder
- ½ teaspoon ground cumin
- ½ teaspoon cayenne pepper

How to Prepare
1. Preheat your oven to 425ºF and line a large baking dish with parchment paper.
2. In a bowl, add the chickpeas, oil, and salt, and toss to coat well.
3. Transfer the chickpeas mixture onto the prepared baking dish and spread in a single layer.
4. Roast for about 20–25 minutes, flipping after every 5 minutes.
5. Meanwhile, in a small bowl, mix together the spices.
6. Remove from the oven and place the chickpeas into a bowl.
7. Add the spice mixture and toss to coat well.
8. Serve immediately.

Nutritional Values
- Calories 248
- Total Fat 12.7 g
- Saturated Fat 1.7 g
- Cholesterol 0 mg
- Sodium 356 mg
- Total Carbs 23.6 g
- Fiber 6.1 g
- Sugar 0.8 g
- Protein 10.4 g

Nuts & Seeds Squares

Preparation time: 20 minutes
Cooking time: 5 minutes
Total time: 25 minutes
Servings: 8

Ingredients

- ½ cup hazelnuts, toasted
- ½ cup walnuts, toasted
- ½ cup almonds, toasted
- ½ cup white sesame seeds
- ½ cup pumpkin seeds, shelled
- 1 cup unsweetened dried cherries
- 2 cups unsweetened dried coconut flakes
- ¼ cup coconut oil
- 1/3 cup maple syrup
- ½ teaspoon ground cinnamon
- ½ teaspoon salt

How to Prepare

1. Line a 13x9-inch baking dish with parchment paper. Set aside.
2. In a large bowl, add the hazelnuts, walnuts, and almonds and mix well.
3. Transfer 1 cup of the nut mixture into another large bowl and chop them roughly.
4. In the food processor, add the remaining nut mixture and pulse until finely ground.
5. Now, transfer the ground nut mixture into the bowl of the chopped nuts.
6. Add the seeds and coconut flakes and mix well.
7. In a small pan, add the oil, maple syrup, and cinnamon over medium-low heat and cook for about 3–5 minutes or until it starts to boil, stirring continuously.
8. Remove from the heat and immediately pour over the nut mixture, stirring continuously until well combined.
9. Set aside to cool slightly.
10. Now, place the mixture into the prepared baking dish evenly and with the back of a spoon, smooth the top surface by pressing slightly.
11. Refrigerate for about 1 hour or until set completely.
12. Remove from refrigerator and cut into equal sized squares and serve.

Nutritional Values

- Calories 496
- Total Fat 41.7 g
- Saturated Fat 22 g
- Cholesterol 0 mg
- Sodium 161 mg
- Total Carbs 24.4 g
- Fiber 7.7 g
- Sugar 12 g
- Protein 9.8 g

Seed Bars

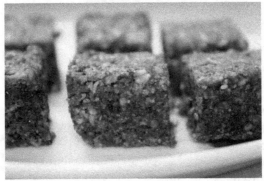

Preparation time: 15 minutes
Total time: 15 minutes
Servings: 10

Ingredients
- 1¼ cups creamy salted peanut butter
- 5 Medjool dates, pitted
- ½ cup unsweetened vegan protein powder
- 2/3 cup hemp seeds
- 1/3 cup chia seeds

How to Prepare
1. Line a loaf pan with parchment paper. Set aside.
2. In a food processor, add the peanut butter and dates and pulse until well combined.
3. Add the protein powder, hemp seeds, and chia seeds and pulse until well combined.
4. Now, place the mixture into the prepared loaf pan and with the back of a spoon, smooth the top surface.
5. Freeze for at least 10–15 minutes, or until set.
6. Cut into 10 equal sized bars and serve.

Nutritional Values
- Calories 308
- Total Fat 21.2 g
- Saturated Fat 1.8 g
- Cholesterol 0 mg
- Sodium 123 mg
- Total Carbs 17.1 g
- Fiber 6.5 g
- Sugar 9.7 g
- Protein 16 g

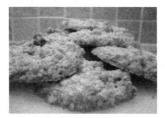

Oatmeal Cookies

Preparation time: 15 minutes
Cooking time: 14 minutes
Total time: 29 minutes
Servings: 6

Ingredients
- 2 medium ripe bananas, peeled
- 1 cup old fashioned oats
- 2 scoops unsweetened vegan protein powder
- 2 tablespoons unsalted peanut butter
- 2 tablespoons vegan mini chocolate chips

How to Prepare
1. Preheat the oven to 350ºF and line a large baking sheet with greased parchment paper.
2. In a bowl, add bananas and with a fork, mash well.
3. Add the oats, whey protein powder, and peanut butter, and mix until well combined.
4. Gently, fold in the chocolate chips.
5. Spoon the mixture onto prepared cookie sheet in a single layer and with your finger, flatten each cookie slightly.
6. Bake for about 12–14 minutes or until golden-brown.
7. Remove from oven and place the cookie sheet onto a wire rack to cool for about 5 minutes.
8. Now, invert the cookies onto the wire rack to cool before serving.

Nutritional Values
- Calories 242
- Total Fat 7.6 g
- Saturated 2.6 g
- Cholesterol 0 mg
- Sodium 115 mg
- Total Carbs 29.1 g
- Fiber 4.6 g
- Sugar 6 g
- Protein 14.2 g

NUTRIENT-PACKED PROTEIN SALAD RECIPES

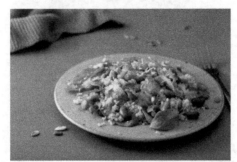

Quinoa & Chickpea Salad

Preparation time: 20 minutes
Total time: 20 minutes
Servings: 4

Ingredients
- 2 cups cooked quinoa
- 1½ cups canned red kidney beans, rinsed and drained
- 3 cups fresh baby spinach
- ¼ cup sun-dried tomatoes, chopped
- ¼ cup fresh dill
- ¼ cup fresh parsley
- ½ cup sunflower seeds
- ¼ cup walnuts, chopped
- 3 tablespoons fresh lemon juice
- Salt and ground black pepper, as required

How to Prepare
1. In a large bowl, add all the ingredients and toss to coat well.
2. Serve immediately.

Nutritional Values
- Calories 489
- Total Fat 13.1 g
- Saturated Fat 1.2 g
- Cholesterol 0 mg
- Sodium 84 mg
- Total Carbs 73.4 g
- Fiber 15.7 g
- Sugar 0.9 g
- Protein 22.7 g

Mixed Grain Salad

Preparation time: 20 minutes
Total time: 20 minutes
Servings: 6

Ingredients

Dressing
- ¼ cup fresh lime juice
- 2 tablespoons maple syrup
- 1 tablespoon Dijon mustard
- ½ teaspoon ground cumin
- 1 teaspoon garlic powder
- Salt and ground black pepper, to taste
- ½ cup extra-virgin olive oil

Salad
- 2 cups fresh mango, peeled, pitted, and cubed
- 2 tablespoon fresh lime juice, divided
- 2 avocados, peeled, pitted, and cubed
- Pinch of salt
- 1 cup cooked quinoa
- 2 (14-ounce) cans black beans, rinsed and drained
- 1 (15¼-ounce) can corn, rinsed and drained
- 1 small red onion, chopped
- 1 jalapeño, seeded and chopped finely
- ½ cup fresh cilantro, chopped
- 6 cups romaine lettuce, shredded

How to Prepare

1. For dressing: in a blender, add all the ingredients (except oil) and pulse until well combined.
2. While the motor is running, gradually add the oil and pulse until smooth.
3. For salad: in a bowl, add the mango and 1 tablespoon of lime juice and toss to coat well.
4. In another bowl, add the avocado, a pinch of salt, and remaining lime juice and toss to coat well.
5. In a large serving bowl, add the mango, avocado, and remaining salad ingredients and mix.
6. Place the dressing and toss to coat well.
7. Serve immediately.

Nutritional Values

- Calories 631
- Total Fat 33.6 g
- Saturated Fat 5.5 g
- Cholesterol 0 mg
- Sodium 100 mg
- Total Carbs 73 g
- Fiber 16.4 g
- Sugar 15.2 g
- Protein 15.9 g

Rice & Tofu Salad

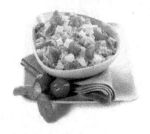

Preparation time: 15 minutes
Total time: 15 minutes
Servings: 4

Ingredients

Salad
- 1 (12-ounce) package firm tofu, pressed, drained, and sliced
- 1½ cups cooked brown rice
- 3 large tomatoes, peeled and chopped
- ¼ cup fresh basil leaves

Dressing
- 3 scallions, chopped
- 2 tablespoons black sesame seeds, toasted
- 2 tablespoons low-sodium soy sauce
- ½ teaspoon sesame oil, toasted
- Drop of hot pepper sauce
- 1 tablespoon maple syrup
- ¼ teaspoon red chili powder

How to Prepare

1. In a large serving bowl, place all the ingredients and toss to coat well.
2. Serve immediately.

Nutritional Values
- Calories 393
- Total Fat 8.6 g
- Saturated Fat 1.5 g
- Cholesterol 0 mg
- Sodium 464 mg
- Total Carbs 66.9 g
- Fiber 5.7 g
- Sugar 7.9 g
- Protein 15.1 g

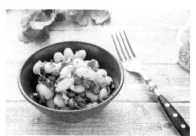

Kidney Bean & Pomegranate Salad

Preparation time: 15 minutes
Total time: 15 minutes
Servings: 3

Ingredients
- 2 cups canned white kidney beans, rinsed and drained
- 1 cup fresh pomegranate seeds
- 1/3 cup scallion (green part), chopped finely
- 2 tablespoons fresh parsley, chopped
- 1 tablespoon fresh lime juice
- Salt and ground black pepper, as required

How to Prepare
1. In a large serving bowl, place all the ingredients and toss to coat well.
2. Serve immediately.

Nutritional Values
- Calories 180
- Total Fat 0 g
- Saturated Fat 0 g
- Cholesterol 0 mg
- Sodium 74 mg
- Total Carbs 35 g
- Fiber 14.1 g
- Sugar 5.3 g
- Protein 12 g

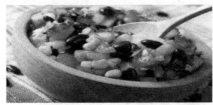

Bean & Corn Salad

Preparation time: 15 minutes
Total time: 15 minutes
Servings: 8

Ingredients
Salad
- 1 (10-ounce) package frozen corn kernels, thawed
- 3 (15-ounce) cans black beans, rinsed and drained
- 2 large red bell peppers, seeded and chopped
- 1 large red onion, chopped

Dressing
- ¼ cup fresh cilantro, minced
- 1 garlic clove, minced
- 1 tablespoon maple syrup
- ½ cup balsamic vinegar
- ½ cup olive oil
- 1 tablespoon fresh lime juice
- 1 tablespoon fresh lemon juice
- ½ teaspoon red pepper flakes, crushed
- Salt and ground black pepper, as required

How to Prepare
1. For salad: add all the ingredients in a large serving bowl and mix well.
2. For dressing: add all the ingredients in a bowl and beat until well combined.
3. Place the dressing over salad and gently toss to coat well.
4. Serve immediately.

Nutritional Values
- Calories 310
- Total Fat 14.3 g
- Saturated Fat 1.9 g
- Cholesterol 0 mg
- Sodium 43 mg
- Total Carbs 36.5 g
- Fiber 9.5 g
- Sugar 5 g
- Protein 10.7 g

Pasta & Veggie Salad

Preparation time: 25 minutes
Cooking time: 10 minutes
Total time: 35 minutes
Servings: 6

Ingredients

Salad
- 12 ounces whole-wheat pasta
- 2 cups carrot, peeled and chopped
- 1 cup black olives, pitted and sliced
- 1 cup red bell pepper, seeded and chopped
- 1 cup yellow bell pepper, seeded and chopped
- 1 cup orange bell pepper, seeded and chopped
- ¾ cup fresh cilantro, chopped
- 1 jalapeño pepper, seeded and chopped finely
- 1 cup scallions, chopped

Vinaigrette
- 2 tablespoons balsamic vinegar
- 2 tablespoons extra-virgin olive oil
- 1 tablespoon fresh lemon juice
- 1 teaspoon sesame oil
- 1½ teaspoons red pepper flakes, crushed

How to Prepare

1. In a pan of salted boiling water, add the pasta and cook for about 8–10 minutes or according to the package's directions.
2. Drain the pasta well and rinse under cold water.
3. Transfer the pasta into a large bowl.
4. Meanwhile, in another pan of salted boiling water, add the edamame and cook for about 5 minutes.
5. Drain the edamame well.
6. In the bowl of pasta, add the edamame and remaining salad ingredients (except scallions) and gently stir to combine.
7. For vinaigrette: in another bowl, add all the ingredients and beat until well combined.
8. Pour the vinaigrette over salad and gently stir to combine.
9. Serve immediately with the garnishing of scallion and sesame seeds.

Nutritional Values
- Calories 333
- Total Fat 9.4 g
- Saturated Fat 1.2 g
- Cholesterol 0 mg
- Sodium 232 mg
- Total Carbs 54.5 g
- Fiber 5.5 g
- Sugar 5.5 g
- Protein 10 g

Chickpea & Veggie Salad

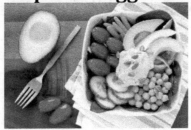

Preparation time: 20 minutes
Total time: 20 minutes
Servings: 2

Ingredients
- 1 medium avocado, peeled, pitted, and sliced
- 2 teaspoons fresh lime juice
- 2 cups fresh baby spinach
- ¾ cup boiled chickpeas
- 1 cup grape tomatoes
- 1 cup baby carrots
- 1 medium cucumber, sliced
- ¼ cup red onion, sliced
- 2 tablespoons olive oil
- 6 tablespoons hummus
- 2 tablespoons pumpkin seeds

How to Prepare
1. In a bowl, add the avocado slices and lemon juice and toss to coat well.
2. In the bottom of 2 serving bowls, divide the spinach and top with the chickpeas, vegetables, and avocado slices.
3. Drizzle each bowl with oil and top with hummus.
4. Garnish with pumpkin seeds and serve immediately.

Nutritional Values
- Calories 611
- Total Fat 43.6 g
- Saturated Fat 7.6 g
- Cholesterol 0 mg
- Sodium 764 mg
- Total Carbs 49.1 g
- Fiber 19.9 g
- Sugar 12 g
- Protein 14.6 g

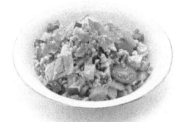

Farro & Veggie Salad

Preparation time: 15 minutes
Total time: 15 minutes
Servings: 3

Ingredients
- 6 teaspoons extra-virgin olive oil
- 2 teaspoons balsamic vinegar
- Salt and ground black pepper, to taste
- 2 cups cooked farro
- 1 cup carrots, peeled and sliced
- 1 cup yellow bell pepper, seeded and chopped
- 1 cup grape tomatoes, halved
- 1 cup cucumber, chopped
- 2 tablespoons fresh cilantro leaves

How to Prepare
1. In a small bowl, add oil, vinegar, salt, and black pepper, and beat until well combined.
2. In a large bowl, add the remaining ingredients and mix well.
3. Pour the vinaigrette over salad and toss to coat well.
4. Serve immediately.

Nutritional Values
- Calories 551
- Total Fat 9.6 g
- Saturated Fat 1.4 g
- Cholesterol 0 mg
- Sodium 161 mg
- Total Carbs 98 g
- Fiber 10.4 g
- Sugar 6 g
- Protein 20.1 g

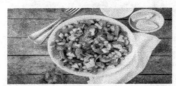

Chickpea & Veggie Salad

Preparation time: 20 minutes
Total time: 20 minutes
Servings: 4

Ingredients
Salad
- 18 ounces canned chickpeas, drained and rinsed
- 2 large avocados, peeled, pitted, and chopped
- 2 cups cucumber, chopped
- 2 cups cherry tomatoes, halved
- 6 cups fresh baby spinach
- 4 tablespoons fresh parsley leaves, chopped

Dressing
- 1 serrano pepper, seeded and minced
- 1 garlic clove, minced
- ¼ cup extra-virgin olive oil
- 3 tablespoons balsamic vinegar
- 1 tablespoon fresh lemon juice
- ¼ teaspoon red pepper flakes, crushed
- Salt and ground black pepper, as required

How to Prepare
1. For salad: in a large serving bowl, add all the ingredients and mix.
2. For dressing: in another bowl, add all the ingredients and beat till well combined.
3. Pour dressing over salad and gently toss to coat well.
4. Serve immediately.

Nutritional Values
- Calories 473
- Total Fat 32.1 g
- Saturated Fat 5.7 g
- Cholesterol 0 mg
- Sodium 122 mg
- Total Carbs 37.1 g
- Fiber 14.1 g
- Sugar 3.9 g
- Protein 12.6 g

Bean & Couscous Salad

Preparation time: 20 minutes
Cooking time: 5 minutes
Total time: 25 minutes
Servings: 4

Ingredients
Salad
- ½ cup homemade vegetable broth
- ½ cup couscous
- 1 cup frozen corn, thawed
- 3 cups canned red kidney beans, rinsed and drained
- 2 large tomatoes, chopped
- 6 cups fresh spinach, torn

Dressing
- 1 garlic clove, minced
- 2 tablespoons shallots, minced
- 2 teaspoons lemon zest, grated finely
- ¼ cup fresh lemon juice
- 2 tablespoons extra-virgin olive oil
- Salt and ground black pepper, to taste

How to Prepare
1. In a pan, add the broth over medium heat and bring to a boil.
2. Add the couscous and stir to combine.
3. Cover the pan and immediately remove from the heat.
4. Set aside, covered for about 5–10 minutes, or until all the liquid is absorbed.
5. For salad: in a large serving bowl, add the couscous and remaining ingredients and stir to combine.
6. For dressing: in another small bowl, add all the ingredients and beat until well combined.
7. Pour the dressing over salad and gently toss to coat well.
8. Serve immediately.

Nutritional Values
- Calories 365
- Total Fat 8.3 g
- Saturated Fat 1.3 g
- Cholesterol 0 mg
- Sodium 208 mg
- Total Carbs 57.9 g
- Fiber 19.3 g
- Sugar 4.3 g
- Protein 19.1 g

STAPLE LUNCH RECIPES

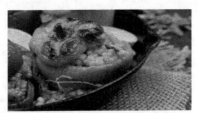

Couscous-Stuffed Bell Peppers

Preparation time: 15 minutes
Cooking time: 40 minutes
Total time: 55 minutes
Servings: 4

Ingredients
- 1 cup water
- ½ cup uncooked couscous
- 4 bell peppers, tops removed and seeded
- 2 tablespoons fresh parsley, chopped
- 1 tablespoon olive oil
- 1 tablespoon fresh lemon juice
- Salt and freshly ground black pepper, to taste

How to Prepare
1. In a pan, add the water over medium-high heat and bring to a rolling boil.
2. Stir in the couscous and immediately cover the pan.
3. Remove from the heat and set the pan aside, covered for about 10 minutes.
4. With a fork, fluff the couscous and let it cool completely.
5. Preheat the oven to 350ºF. Lightly grease a baking sheet.
6. Arrange the bell peppers onto the prepared baking sheet.
7. In a large bowl, add the cooled couscous and remaining ingredients and mix until well combined.
8. Stuff each bell pepper with couscous mixture.
9. Bake for about 35 minutes or until bell peppers are tender.

Nutritional Values
- Calories 151
- Total Fat 4 g
- Saturated Fat 0.6 g
- Cholesterol 0 mg
- Sodium 48 mg
- Total Carbs 26 g
- Fiber 2.8 g
- Sugar 6.1 g
- Protein 4.1 g

Pasta with Asparagus

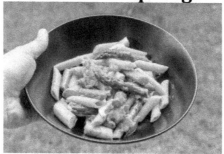

Preparation time: 15 minutes
Cooking time: 12 minutes
Total time: 27 minutes
Servings: 4

Ingredients
- ¼ cup olive oil
- 5 garlic cloves, minced
- ½ teaspoon red pepper flakes, crushed
- 1/8 teaspoon hot pepper sauce
- 1 pound asparagus, trimmed and cut into 1½-inch pieces
- Salt and ground black pepper, to taste
- ½ pound cooked whole-wheat pasta, drained

How to Prepare
1. In a large cast-iron skillet, heat the oil over medium heat and cook the garlic, red pepper flakes, and hot pepper sauce for about 1 minute.
2. Add the asparagus, salt, and black pepper and cook for about 8–10 minutes, stirring occasionally.
3. Place the hot pasta and toss to coat well.
4. Serve immediately.

Nutritional Values
- Calories 326
- Total Fat 13.8 g
- Saturated Fat 1.9 g
- Cholesterol 0 mg
- Sodium 52 mg
- Total Carbs 39 g
- Fiber 8.5 g
- Sugar 2.2 g
- Protein 11.9 g

Black-Eyed Peas Curry

Preparation time: 15 minutes
Cooking time: 1 hour 10 minutes
Total time: 1 hour 25 minutes
Servings: 4

Ingredients
- 2 tablespoons canola oil
- 1 medium onion, chopped
- ¼ cup shallot, chopped
- 3 cups tomatoes, chopped finely
- 2 fresh green chilies, chopped finely
- 1 teaspoon red chili powder
- 1 teaspoon ground cumin
- Salt and ground black pepper, to taste
- 16 ounces dried black-eyed peas
- 3 cups water
- 2 tablespoons fresh parsley, chopped

How to Prepare
1. In a large pan, heat the oil over medium heat and sauté the onion for about 4–5 minutes.
2. Add the tomatoes, green chilies, spices, salt, and black pepper, and sauté for about 2–3 minutes.
3. Add the black-eyed peas and water and bring to a boil.
4. Reduce the heat to medium-low and cook, covered for about 45–60 minutes.
5. Stir in the lime juice, salt, and black pepper and cook for about 1 minute.
6. Serve hot with the garnishing of parsley.

Nutritional Values
- Calories 193
- Total Fat 8.5 g
- Saturated Fat 0.6 g
- Cholesterol 0 mg
- Sodium 85 mg
- Total Carbs 25.2 g
- Fiber 6.3 g
- Sugar 4.8 g
- Protein 8 g

Lentil Falafel Bowls

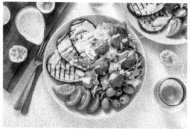

Preparation time: 25 minutes
Cooking time: 20 minutes
Total time: 45 minutes
Servings: 4

Ingredients
Falafel
- 4 tablespoons fresh parsley
- 1 small red onion, chopped roughly
- 2 garlic cloves, peeled
- 1 cup red lentils, soaked overnight
- 2 tablespoons chickpea flour
- 2 tablespoons fresh lemon juice
- 2 tablespoons olive oil
- ½ teaspoon ground cumin
- Salt and ground black pepper, to taste

Eggplant
- 1 large eggplant
- 2 tablespoons olive oil
- Salt and freshly ground black pepper, to taste

Salad
- 1 cup green olives, pitted
- 2 large tomatoes, sliced
- 2 cups fresh baby greens

Dressing
- ¼ cup tahini
- 2 garlic cloves, minced
- 2 tablespoons fresh lemon juice
- 1 tablespoon white miso
- ¼ cup water

How to Prepare
1. Preheat the oven to 400°F and line a baking sheet with parchment paper.
2. For falafel: in a food processor, add the parsley, onion, and garlic, and pulse until finely chopped.
3. Now, place the remaining ingredients and pulse until just combined.

4. Make small-sized patties from the mixture.
5. Arrange the patties onto the prepared baking sheet in a single layer.
6. Bake for about 18–20 minutes, or until patties become golden-brown.
7. Meanwhile, for eggplant: preheat grill to medium-high heat. Grease the grill grate.
8. Carefully, cut the stem end off of the eggplant.
9. Then, cut the eggplant into 1-inch-thick slices lengthwise.
10. Coat the eggplant slices with oil evenly and sprinkle with salt and black pepper.
11. Place the eggplant slices onto the grill grate and cook for about 4–5 minutes per side.
12. For dressing: in a bowl, add all the ingredients and beat until well combined.
13. Divide salad ingredients and falafel patties into serving bowls evenly.
14. Drizzle with dressing and serve immediately.

Nutritional Values
- Calories 513
- Total Fat 27.4 g
- Saturated Fat 3.9 g
- Cholesterol 0 mg
- Sodium 529 mg
- Total Carbs 53 g
- Fiber 24.4 g
- Sugar 9.1 g
- Protein 19.7 g

Buddha Bowl

Preparation time: 20 minutes
Total time: 20 minutes
Servings: 6

Ingredients

Dressing
- ¼ cup balsamic vinegar
- ¼ cup low-sodium soy sauce
- 2 tablespoons water
- 1 teaspoon sesame oil, toasted
- 1 teaspoon Sriracha
- 3–4 drops liquid stevia

Salad
- 3 cups canned chickpeas, rinsed and drained
- 1½ pounds baked firm tofu, cubed
- 2 large zucchinis, sliced thinly
- 2 large yellow bell peppers, seeded and sliced thinly
- 3 cups cherry tomatoes, halved
- 2 cups radishes, sliced thinly
- 2 cups purple cabbage, shredded
- 6 cups fresh baby spinach
- 2 tablespoons white sesame seeds

How to Prepare

1. For dressing: in a bowl, add all the ingredients and beat until well combined.
2. Divide the chickpeas, tofu, and vegetables into serving bowls.
3. Drizzle with dressing and serve immediately with the garnishing of sesame seeds.

Nutritional Values
- Calories 305
- Total Fat 8.6 g
- Saturated Fat 1.4 g
- Cholesterol 0 mg
- Sodium 696 mg
- Total Carbs 38.4 g
- Fiber 11 g
- Sugar 9.2 g
- Protein 21.4 g

Vegetarian Taco Bowl

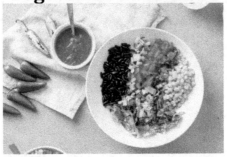

Preparation time: 15 minutes
Total time: 15 minutes
Servings: 2

Ingredients
- 2 teaspoons olive oil
- 1 red bell pepper, seeded and chopped
- 1 red onion, sliced
- 1 cup canned black beans, rinsed and drained
- ½ cup frozen corn, thawed
- 3 cups lettuce, chopped
- 1 jalapeño pepper, seeded and minced
- 1 tablespoon fresh lime juice
- ¼ cup salsa

How to Prepare
1. Divide the beans, corn, veggies, lettuce, and jalapeño pepper into serving bowls.
2. Drizzle with lime juice and serve alongside the salsa.

Nutritional Values
- Calories 257
- Total Fat 6.5 g
- Saturated Fat 0.8 g
- Cholesterol 0 mg
- Sodium 224 mg
- Total Carbs 39.9 g
- Fiber 10.2 g
- Sugar 8.6 g
- Protein 11 g

Tofu & Veggie Burgers

Preparation time: 20 minutes
Cooking time: 8 minutes
Total time: 28 minutes
Servings: 2

Ingredients
Patties
- ½ cup firm tofu, pressed and drained
- 1 medium carrot, peeled and grated
- 1 tablespoon onion, chopped
- 1 tablespoon scallion, chopped
- 1 tablespoon fresh parsley, chopped
- ½ garlic clove, minced
- 2 teaspoons low-sodium soy sauce
- 1 tablespoon cornflour
- 1 teaspoon nutritional yeast flakes
- ½ teaspoon Dijon mustard
- 1 teaspoon paprika
- ¼ teaspoon ground turmeric
- ½ teaspoon ground black pepper
- 2 tablespoons canola oil

For Serving
- 1 small avocado, peeled, pitted, and sliced
- ½ cup cherry tomatoes, halved
- 2 cup fresh baby greens

How to Prepare
1. For patties: in a bowl, add the tofu and with a fork, mash well.
2. Add the remaining ingredients (except for oil) and mix until well combined.
3. Make 4 equal-sized patties from the mixture.
4. Heat the oil in a frying pan over low heat and cook the patties for about 4 minutes per side.
5. Divide the avocado, tomatoes, and greens onto serving plates.
6. Top each plate with 2 patties and serve.

Nutritional Values
- Calories 342
- Total Fat 28.5 g
- Saturated Fat 4 g
- Cholesterol 0 mg
- Sodium 335 mg
- Total Carbs 17.7 g
- Fiber 7.7 g
- Sugar 4.5 g
- Protein 10 g

Buckwheat Burgers

Preparation time: 20 minutes
Cooking time: 45 minutes
Total time: 1 hour 5 minutes
Servings: 2

Ingredients

Patties

- ¾ cup dry buckwheat
- 1½ cups water
- Salt, to taste
- 2 tablespoons olive oil, divided
- ½ of large yellow onion, chopped finely
- ½ of large carrot, peeled and grated
- ½ celery stalk, chopped finely
- 1 fresh kale leaf, tough ribs removed and chopped finely
- 1 large cooked sweet potato, mashed
- 2 tablespoons almond butter
- 2 tablespoons low-sodium soy sauce

For Serving

- 3 cups fresh baby greens
- 1 cup cherry tomatoes, halved
- 1 cup purple cabbage, shredded
- 1 yellow bell pepper, seeded and sliced

How to Prepare

1. Preheat oven to 350ºF and line a baking sheet with parchment paper.
2. For patties: heat a non-stick frying pan over medium heat and toast the buckwheat for about 5 minutes, stirring continuously.
3. Add the water and salt and bring to a boil over high heat.
4. Reduce the heat to low and cook, covered for about 15 minutes or until all the water is absorbed.
5. Meanwhile, heat 1 tablespoon of the oil in a skillet over medium heat and sauté the onion for about 4–5 minutes.
6. Add the carrot and celery and cook for about 5 minutes.
7. Stir in the remaining ingredients and remove from the heat.
8. Transfer the mixture into a bowl with buckwheat and stir to combine.
9. Set aside to cool completely.
10. Make 4 equal-sized patties from the mixture.
11. Arrange the patties onto the prepared baking sheet in a single layer and bake for about 20 minutes per side.
12. Divide the greens, tomatoes, cabbage, and bell pepper onto serving plates.
13. Top each plate with 2 patties and serve

Nutritional Values

- Calories 588
- Total Fat 25.2 g
- Saturated Fat 3.1 g
- Cholesterol 0 mg
- Sodium 1000 mg
- Total Carbs 84.8 g
- Fiber 15.4 g
- Sugar 16.4 g
- Protein 16.7 g

Stuffed Avocados

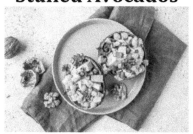

Preparation time: 15 minutes
Total time: 15 minutes
Servings: 2

Ingredients
- 1 large avocado, halved and pitted
- 1 cup cooked chickpeas
- ¼ cup walnuts, chopped
- ¼ cup celery stalks, chopped
- 1 scallion (green part), sliced
- 1 small garlic clove, minced
- 1½ tablespoons fresh lemon juice
- ½ teaspoon olive oil
- Salt and ground black pepper, to taste
- 1 tablespoon sunflower seeds
- 1 tablespoon fresh cilantro, chopped

How to Prepare
1. With a spoon, scoop out the flesh from each avocado half.
2. Then, cut half of the avocado flesh in equal-sized cubes.
3. In a large bowl, add avocado cubes and remaining ingredients except for sunflower seeds and cilantro and toss to coat well.
4. Stuff each avocado half with chickpeas mixture evenly.
5. Serve immediately with the garnishing of sunflower seeds and cilantro.

Nutritional Values
- Calories 440
- Total Fat 32.2 g
- Saturated Fat 5 g
- Cholesterol 0 mg
- Sodium 428 mg
- Total Carbs 30.2 g
- Fiber 14.4 g
- Sugar 2.3 g
- Protein 12.6 g

Stuffed Sweet Potatoes

Preparation time: 20 minutes
Cooking time: 40 minutes
Total time: 1 hour
Servings: 2

Ingredients

Sweet Potatoes
- 1large sweet potato, halved
- ½ tablespoonolive oil
- Salt and ground black pepper, to taste

Filling
- ½ tablespoonolive oil
- 1/3 cup canned chickpeas, rinsed and drained
- 1 teaspoon curry powder
- 1/8 teaspoongarlic powder
- 1/3 cup cooked quinoa
- Salt and ground black pepper, to taste
- 1 teaspoon fresh lime juice
- 1 teaspoon fresh cilantro, chopped
- 1 teaspoon sesame seeds

How to Prepare

1. Preheat the oven to 375ºF.
2. Rub each sweet potato half with oil evenly.
3. Arrange the sweet potato halves onto a baking sheet, cut-side down, and sprinkle with salt and black pepper.
4. Bake for 40 minutes, or until sweet potato becomes tender.
5. Meanwhile, for filling: in a skillet, heat the oil over medium heat and cook the chickpeas, curry powder, and garlic powder for about 6–8 minutes, stirring frequently.
6. Stir in the cooked quinoa, salt, and black pepper, and remove from the heat.
7. Remove from the oven and arrange each sweet potato halves onto a plate.
8. With a fork, fluff the flesh of each half slightly.
9. Place chickpea mixture in each half and drizzle with lime juice
10. Serve immediately with the garnishing of cilantro and sesame seeds.

Nutritional Values
- Calories 340
- Total Fat 8.2 g
- Saturated Fat 1.1 g
- Cholesterol 0 mg
- Sodium 117 mg
- Total Carbs 50 g
- Fiber 10 g
- Sugar 8.8 g
- Protein 12.6 g

WHOLE FOOD LUNCH & DINNER RECIPES
Cauliflower with Peas

Preparation time: 15 minutes
Cooking time: 15 minutes
Total time: 30 minutes
Servings: 3

Ingredients

- 2 medium tomatoes, chopped
- ¼ cup water
- 2 tablespoons olive oil
- 3 garlic cloves, minced
- ½ tablespoon fresh ginger, minced
- 1 teaspoon ground cumin
- 2 teaspoons ground coriander
- 1 teaspoon cayenne pepper
- ¼ teaspoon ground turmeric
- 2 cups cauliflower, chopped
- 1 cup fresh green peas, shelled
- Salt and ground black pepper, to taste
- ½ cup warm water

How to Prepare

1. In a blender, add tomato and ¼ cup of water and pulse until a smooth puree forms. Set aside.
2. In a large skillet, heat the oil over medium heat and sauté the garlic, ginger, green chilies, and spices for about 1 minute.
3. Add the cauliflower, peas, and tomato puree and cook, stirring for about 3–4 minutes.
4. Add the warm water and bring to a boil.
5. Reduce the heat to medium-low and cook, covered for about 8–10 minutes or until vegetables are done completely.
6. Serve hot.

Nutritional Values

- Calories 163
- Total Fat 10.1 g
- Saturated Fat 1.5 g
- Cholesterol 0 mg
- Sodium 79 mg
- Total Carbs 16.1 g
- Fiber 5.6 g
- Sugar 6.7 g
- Protein 6 g

Burgers with Mushroom Sauce

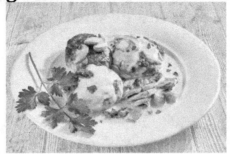

Preparation time: 25 minutes
Cooking time: 30 minutes
Total time: 55 minutes
Servings: 2

Ingredients
Patties
- ½ cup millet, rinsed
- 1 cup hot water
- 1 (14-ounce) can chickpeas, rinsed, drained, and mashed roughly
- 1 carrot, peeled and grated finely
- ½ of red bell pepper, seeded and chopped
- ½ of yellow onion, chopped
- 1 garlic clove, minced
- ½ tablespoon fresh cilantro, chopped
- ½ teaspoon curry powder
- Salt and ground black pepper, to taste
- 4 tablespoons chickpea flour
- 2 tablespoons canola oil

Mushroom Sauce
- 2 cups unsweetened soymilk
- 2 tablespoons arrowroot flour
- 1 tablespoon low-sodium soy sauce
- Pinch of ground black pepper
- 1 teaspoon olive oil
- ¾ cup fresh button mushrooms, chopped
- 1 garlic clove, minced
- 2 tablespoons fresh chives, chopped

How to Prepare
1. For patties: heat a small non-stick pan over medium heat and toast the millet for about 5 minutes, stirring continuously.
2. Add the hot water and bring to a rolling boil.
3. Reduce the heat to low and simmer, covered for about 15 minutes.

4. Remove from the heat and set aside, covered for about 10 minutes.
5. Uncover the pan and let the millet cool completely.
6. After cooling, fluff the millet with a fork.
7. In a large bowl, add the millet and remaining ingredients (except for chickpea flour and oil) and mix until well combined.
8. Slowly, add the chickpea flour, 1 tablespoon at a time, and mix well.
9. Make 4 equal-sized patties from the mixture.
10. In a non-stick frying pan, heat the oil over medium heat and cook the patties for about 3–4 minutes per side, or until golden-brown.
11. Meanwhile, for mushroom sauce: in a bowl, add the soymilk, flour, soy sauce, and black pepper and beat until smooth. Set aside.
12. Heat the oil in a skillet over medium heat and sauté the mushrooms and garlic for about 3 minutes.
13. Stir in the soymilk mixture and cook for about 8 minutes, stirring frequently.
14. Stir in the chives and remove from the heat.
15. Place 2 patties onto each serving plate and top with mushroom sauce.
16. Serve immediately.

Nutritional Values
- Calories 713
- Total Fat 24.2 g
- Saturated Fat 2.3 g
- Cholesterol 0 mg
- Sodium 674 mg
- Total Carbs 92 g
- Fiber 17.1 g
- Sugar 8.5 g
- Protein 29.5 g

Rice & Lentil Loaf

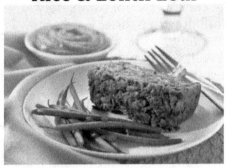

Preparation time: 20 minutes
Cooking time: 1 hour 50 minutes
Total time: 2 hours 10 minutes
Servings: 6

Ingredients
- 1¾ cups plus 2 tablespoons water, divided
- ½ cup wild rice
- ½ cup brown lentils
- Salt, to taste
- ½ teaspoon Italian seasoning
- 1 medium yellow onion, chopped
- 1 celery stalk, chopped
- 6 cremini mushrooms, chopped
- 4 garlic cloves, minced
- ¾ cup rolled oats
- ½ cup walnuts, chopped finely
- ¾ cup sugar-free ketchup
- ½ teaspoon red pepper flakes, crushed
- 1 teaspoon fresh rosemary, minced
- 2 teaspoons fresh thyme, minced

How to Prepare
1. In a pan, add 1¾ cups of the water, rice, lentils, salt, and Italian seasoning over medium-high heat and bring to a rolling boil.
2. Reduce the heat to low and cook, covered for about 45 minutes.
3. Remove the pan from heat and set aside, covered for at least 10 minutes.
4. Preheat your oven to 350°F and line a 9x5-inch loaf pan with parchment paper.
5. In a skillet, heat the remaining water over medium heat and sauté the onion, celery, mushrooms, and garlic for about 4–5 minutes.
6. Remove from the heat and set aside to cool slightly.
7. In a large bowl, add the oats, walnuts, ketchup, and fresh herbs and mix until well combined.
8. Add the rice mixture and vegetable mixture and mix well.

9. In a blender, add the mixture and pulse until just a chunky mixture forms.
10. Place the mixture into the prepared loaf pan evenly.
11. With a piece of foil, cover the loaf pan and bake for about 40 minutes.
12. Uncover and bake for 20 minutes more, or until top becomes golden-brown.
13. Remove from the oven and place the loaf pan onto a wire rack for about 10 minutes.
14. Carefully, invert the loaf onto a platter.
15. Cut into desired sized slices and serve.

Nutritional Values
- Calories 254
- Total Fat 7.5 g
- Saturated Fat 0.6 g
- Cholesterol 0 mg
- Sodium 269 mg
- Total Carbs 38.6 g
- Fiber 8.5 g
- Sugar 8.9 g
- Protein 11.5 g

Chickpeas with Swiss Chard

Preparation time: 15 minutes
Cooking time: 15 minutes
Total time: 30 minutes
Servings: 4

Ingredients
- 2 tablespoons olive oil
- 1 medium yellow onion, chopped
- 4 garlic cloves, minced
- 1 teaspoon dried thyme, crushed
- 1 teaspoon dried oregano, crushed
- ½ teaspoon paprika
- 1 cup tomato, chopped finely
- 2½ cups canned chickpeas, rinsed and drained
- 5 cups Swiss chard
- 2 tablespoons water
- 2 tablespoons fresh lemon juice
- Salt and ground black pepper, to taste
- 3 tablespoons fresh basil, chopped

How to Prepare
1. Heat the olive oil in a skillet over medium heat and sauté onion for about 6-8 minutes.
2. Add the garlic, herbs, and paprika and sauté for about 1 minute.
3. Add the Swiss chard and 2 tablespoons water and cook for about 2-3 minutes.
4. Add the tomatoes and chickpeas and cook for about 2-3 minutes.
5. Add in the lemon juice, salt, and black pepper, and remove from the heat.
6. Serve hot with the garnishing of basil.

Nutritional Values
- Calories 260
- Total Fat 8.6 g
- Saturated Fat 1.1 g
- Cholesterol 0 mg
- Sodium 178 mg
- Total Carbs 34 g
- Fiber 8.6 g
- Sugar 3.1 g
- Protein 12 g

Spicy Black Beans

Preparation time: 15 minutes
Cooking time: 1 hour 25 minutes
Total time: 1 hour 40 minutes
Servings: 5

Ingredients
- 4 cups water
- 1½ cups dried black beans, soaked for 8 hours and drained
- ½ teaspoon ground turmeric
- 3 tablespoons olive oil
- 1 small red onion, chopped finely
- 1 green chili, chopped
- 1 (1-inch) piece fresh ginger, minced
- 2 garlic cloves, minced
- 1½ tablespoons ground coriander
- 1 teaspoon ground cumin
- ½ teaspoon cayenne pepper
- Salt, to taste
- 2 medium tomatoes, chopped finely
- ¼ cup coconut cream
- ½ cup fresh cilantro, chopped

How to Prepare
1. In a large pan, add water, black beans, and turmeric, and bring to a boil on high heat.
2. Now, reduce the heat to low and cook, covered for about 1 hour or until desired doneness of beans.
3. Meanwhile, in a skillet, heat the oil over medium heat and sauté the onion for about 4–5 minutes.
4. Add the green chili, ginger, garlic, spices, and salt, and sauté for about 1–2 minutes.
5. Stir in the tomatoes and cook for about 10 minutes, stirring occasionally.
6. Transfer the tomato mixture into the pan with black beans and stir to combine.
7. Reduce the heat to medium-low and cook for about 20–25 minutes.
8. Serve hot with the garnishing of coconut cream and cilantro.

Nutritional Values
- Calories 344
- Total Fat 11.9 g
- Saturated Fat 3.8 g
- Cholesterol 0 mg
- Sodium 50 mg
- Total Carbs 48.5 g
- Fiber 10 g
- Sugar 10.8 g
- Protein 13.6 g

Mixed Bean Soup

Preparation time: 20 minutes
Cooking time: 45 minutes
Total time: 1 hour 5 minutes
Servings: 12

Ingredients
- ¼ cup vegetable oil
- 1 large onion, chopped
- 1 large sweet potato, peeled and cubed
- 3 carrots, peeled and chopped
- 3 celery stalks, chopped
- 3 garlic cloves, minced
- 2 teaspoons dried thyme, crushed
- 1 (4-ounce) can green chilies
- 2 jalapeño peppers, chopped
- 1 tablespoon ground cumin
- 4 large tomatoes, chopped finely
- 2 (16-ounce) cans great northern beans, rinsed and drained
- 2 (15¼-ounce) cans red kidney beans, rinsed and drained
- 1 (15-ounce) can black beans, drained and rinsed
- 9 cups homemade vegetable broth
- 1 cup fresh cilantro, chopped

How to Prepare
1. In a Dutch oven, heat the oil over medium heat and sauté the onion, sweet potato, carrots, and celery for about 6–8 minutes.
2. Add the garlic, thyme, green chilies, jalapeño peppers, and cumin and sauté for about 1 minute.
3. Add in the tomatoes and cook for about 2–3 minutes.
4. Add the beans and broth and bring to a boil over medium-high heat.
5. Cover the pan with lid and cook for about 25–30 minutes.
6. Stir in the cilantro and remove from heat.
7. Serve hot.

Nutritional Values
- Calories 563
- Total Fat 6.8 g
- Saturated Fat 1.4 g
- Cholesterol 0 mg
- Sodium 528 mg
- Total Carbs 90 g
- Fiber 31.5 g
- Sugar 11 g
- Protein 32.4 g

Barley & Lentil Stew

Preparation time: 20 minutes
Cooking time: 50 minutes
Total time: 1 hour 10 minutes
Servings: 8

Ingredients
- 2 tablespoons olive oil
- 2 carrots, peeled and chopped
- 1 large red onion, chopped
- 2 celery stalks, chopped
- 2 garlic cloves, minced
- 1 teaspoon ground coriander
- 2 teaspoons ground cumin
- 1 teaspoon cayenne pepper
- 1 cup barley
- 1 cup red lentils
- 5 cups tomatoes, chopped finely
- 5-6 cups homemade vegetable broth
- 6 cups fresh spinach, torn
- Salt and ground black pepper, to taste

How to Prepare
1. In a large pan, heat the oil over medium heat and sauté the carrots, onion, and celery for about 5 minutes.
2. Add the garlic and spices and sauté for about 1 minute.
3. Add the barley, lentils, tomatoes, and broth and bring to a rolling boil.
4. Reduce the heat to low and simmer, covered for about 40 minutes.
5. Stir in the spinach, salt, and black pepper, and simmer for about 3-4 minutes.
6. Serve hot.

Nutritional Values
- Calories 264
- Total Fat 5.8 g
- Saturated Fat 1 g
- Cholesterol 0 mg
- Sodium 540 mg
- Total Carbs 41.1 g
- Fiber 14.1 g
- Sugar 5.8 g
- Protein 14.3 g

Chickpea & Pasta Curry

Preparation time: 15 minutes
Cooking time: 40 minutes
Total time: 55 minutes
Servings: 5

Ingredients
- 10 ounces whole-wheat pasta
- 1 tablespoon vegetable oil
- 1 medium white onion, chopped
- 3 garlic cloves, minced
- 1 teaspoon dried basil, crushed
- 1 tablespoon curry powder
- ¼ teaspoon red pepper flakes, crushed
- 2 pounds ripe tomatoes, chopped
- 4 cups cauliflower, cut into bite-sized pieces
- 1 medium red bell pepper, seeded and sliced thinly
- 1 cup water
- ½ cup black raisins
- 1 (15-ounce) can chickpeas, drained and rinsed
- 1 cup fresh baby spinach
- ¼ cup fresh parsley, chopped
- Salt, to taste

How to Prepare
1. In a pan of the salted boiling water, add the pasta and cook for about 8–10 minutes, or according to the package's directions.
2. Drain the pasta well and set aside.
3. Heat the oil in a large cast-iron skillet over medium heat and sauté the onion for about 4–5 minutes.
4. Add the garlic, basil, curry powder, and red pepper flakes and sauté for about 1 minute.
5. Stir in the tomatoes, cauliflower, bell pepper, and water, and bring to a gentle boil.
6. Reduce the heat to medium-low and simmer, covered for about 15–20 minutes.
7. Stir in the raisins and chickpeas and cook for about 5 minutes.
8. Add the spinach and cook for about 3–4 minutes.
9. Stir in the pasta and remove from the heat.
10. Serve hot.

Nutritional Values
- Calories 450
- Total Fat 5.3 g
- Saturated Fat 0.6 g
- Cholesterol 0 mg
- Sodium 102 mg
- Total Carbs 85 g
- Fiber 11.7 g
- Sugar 17.5 g
- Protein 17.7 g

3-Bean Chili

Preparation time: 15 minutes
Cooking time: 1 hour
Total time: 1¼ hours
Servings: 6

Ingredients
- 2 tablespoons olive oil
- 1 green bell pepper, seeded and chopped
- 2 celery stalks, chopped
- 1 scallion, chopped
- 3 garlic cloves, minced
- 1 teaspoon dried oregano, crushed
- 1 tablespoon red chili powder
- 2 teaspoons ground cumin
- 1 teaspoon red pepper flakes, crushed
- 1 teaspoon paprika
- 1 teaspoon ground turmeric
- 1 teaspoon onion powder
- 1 teaspoon garlic powder
- Salt and ground black pepper, to taste
- 4½ cups tomatoes, chopped finely
- 4 cups water
- 1 (16-ounce) can red kidney beans, rinsed and drained
- 1 (16-ounce) can cannellini beans, rinsed and drained
- ½ of (16-ounce) can black beans, rinsed and drained
- 1 jalapeño pepper, seeded and chopped

How to Prepare
1. In a large pan, heat oil over medium heat and cook the bell peppers, celery, scallion, and garlic for about 8–10 minutes, stirring frequently.
2. Add the oregano, spices, salt, black pepper, tomatoes, and water, and bring to a boil.
3. Simmer for about 20 minutes.
4. Stir in the beans and jalapeño pepper and simmer for about 30 minutes.
5. Serve hot.

Nutritional Values
- Calories 342
- Total Fat 6.1 g
- Saturated Fat 0.9 g
- Cholesterol 0 mg
- Sodium 79 mg
- Total Carbs 56 g
- Fiber 21.3 g
- Sugar 6 g
- Protein 20.3 g

Rice Paella

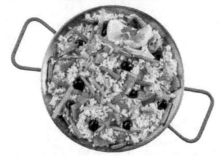

Preparation time: 20 minutes
Cooking time: 20 minutes
Total time: 40 minutes
Servings: 4

Ingredients
- 1cup brown rice
- Pinch of saffron
- 3 tablespoons warm water
- 6cupshomemade vegetable broth
- 1tablespoonolive oil
- 1large yellow onion, chopped
- 1medium green bell pepper, seeded and sliced
- 1medium red bell pepper, seeded and sliced
- 1 cup carrot, peeled and sliced thinly lengthwise
- 4garlic cloves, sliced thinly
- ¾ cupfresh tomatoes, crushed
- 2tablespoonssugar-free tomato paste
- ½ tablespoonhot paprika
- 2cupsgreen beans, trimmed and halved
- 1cupblack olives, pitted
- ¼ cupfresh parsley, chopped
- Salt and ground black pepper, to taste

How to Prepare
1. In a large pan of salted boiling water, add the rice and cook for about 20 minutes.
2. Drain the rice and set aside.
3. In a small bowl, mix together the saffron threads and warm water. Set aside.
4. In a small pan, add the broth and bring to a gentle simmer.
5. Reduce the heat to low to keep the broth warm.
6. Meanwhile, in a large cast-iron skillet, heat the oil and sauté the onions for about 4–5 minutes.
7. Add the bell peppers, carrots, and garlic slices, and cook for about 7 minutes.

8. Stir in the saffron mixture, tomatoes, tomato paste, paprika, salt, and black pepper, and cook for about 2–3 minutes.
9. Add the green beans and stir to combine.
10. Stir in the cooked rice and broth and bring to a boil.
11. Simmer for about 20 minutes, or until all the liquid is absorbed.
12. Stir in the olives and parsley and cover the pan.
13. Remove from the heat and set aside, covered for about 5–10 minutes before serving.

Nutritional Values
- Calories 377
- Total Fat 11.1 g
- Saturated Fat 1.6 g
- Cholesterol 0 mg
- Sodium 1400 mg
- Total Carbs 60.2 g
- Fiber 9.2 g
- Sugar 10.7 g
- Protein 13.7 g

GRAINS & BEANS RECIPES
Baked Beans

Preparation time: 15 minutes
Cooking time: 50 minutes
Total time: 1 hour 5 minutes
Servings: 4

Ingredients
- 1 tablespoon olive oil
- ½ cup green bell pepper, seeded and chopped
- ½ cup white onion, chopped
- 3 garlic cloves, minced
- Salt, to taste
- 1¼ cups sugar-free tomato sauce
- 5 tablespoons pure maple syrup
- ¼ cup water
- 1 tablespoon liquid smoke
- ¼ cup Worcestershire sauce
- Ground black pepper, to taste
- 2 (14-ounce) cans great northern beans, rinsed and drained

How to Prepare
1. Preheat the oven to 325ºF.
2. In a large cast-iron skillet, heat oil over medium heat and cook the bell pepper, onion, garlic, and a little salt for about 4–5 minutes.
3. Add the remaining ingredients (except the beans) and stir to combine.
4. Add the beans and gently stir to combine.
5. Transfer the skillet into the oven and bake for about 30–45 minutes.
6. Serve hot.

Nutritional Values
- Calories 322
- Total Fat 5.3 g
- Saturated Fat 0.5 g
- Cholesterol 0 mg
- Sodium 683 mg
- Total Carbs 59.1 g
- Fiber 14.8 g
- Sugar 24.1 g
- Protein 10 g

Chickpeas with Veggies

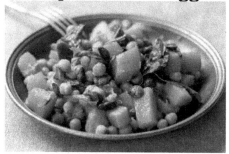

Preparation time: 15 minutes
Cooking time: 35 minutes
Total time: 50 minutes
Servings: 6

Ingredients
- 2 (15-ounce) cans chickpeas, rinsed and drained
- 5 sweet potatoes, peeled and cubed
- 2 tablespoons olive oil
- 1 teaspoon dried basil, crushed
- ½ teaspoon garlic powder
- Salt and ground black pepper, to taste
- 3 cups fresh baby spinach

How to Prepare
1. Preheat the oven to 425ºF. Line a baking dish with parchment paper.
2. In a large bowl, add all ingredients (except for spinach) and toss to coat well. Spread chickpea mixture onto the prepared baking dish in a single layer.
3. Bake for about 30–35 minutes, stirring after every 10 minutes.
4. Remove from the oven and immediately, stir in the spinach.
5. Cover the baking dish for about 5 minutes before serving.

Nutritional Values
- Calories 344
- Total Fat 6.1 g
- Saturated Fat 0.7 g
- Cholesterol 0 mg
- Sodium 100 mg
- Total Carbs 60.1 g
- Fiber 11.4 g
- Sugar 0.8 g
- Protein 11 g

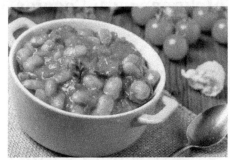

Beans with Salsa

Preparation time: 15 minutes
Cooking time: 11 minutes
Total time: 26 minutes
Servings: 4

Ingredients
- 1 tablespoon canola oil
- 1 small onion, chopped
- 1 garlic clove, minced
- 2 teaspoons fresh cilantro, minced
- 2 (15-ounce) cans pinto beans, rinsed and drained
- 2/3 cup salsa

How to Prepare
1. In a large skillet, heat oil over medium heat and sauté the onion for about 4–5 minutes.
2. Add the garlic and cilantro and sauté for about 1 minute.
3. Stir in the beans and salsa and cook for about 4–5 minutes, or until heated completely.
4. Serve hot.

Nutritional Values
- Calories 329
- Total Fat 4.8 g
- Saturated Fat 0.4 g
- Cholesterol 0 mg
- Sodium 610 mg
- Total Carbs 56.3 g
- Fiber 21.1 g
- Sugar 7.1 g
- Protein 18.7 g

Bean, Corn, & Salsa Chili

Preparation time: 15 minutes
Cooking time: 50 minutes
Total time: 1 hour 5 minutes
Servings: 6

Ingredients
- 1 tablespoon canola oil
- 1 large white onion, chopped finely
- 1 green bell pepper, seeded and chopped finely
- 5 garlic cloves, minced
- 1 teaspoon dried oregano, crushed
- 1½ teaspoons red chili powder
- 1 teaspoon ground cumin
- 2 (15-ounce) cans red kidney beans, rinsed and drained
- 4 cups tomatoes, crushed
- ½ cup mild salsa
- 3 cups frozen corn kernels
- 1 cup homemade vegetable broth
- Salt and ground black pepper, to taste
- ¼ cup fresh cilantro, chopped

How to Prepare
1. In a large pan, heat oil over medium-high heat and sauté the onion and bell pepper for about 5 minutes.
2. Add the garlic, oregano, and spices and sauté for about 1 minute.
3. Add the beans, tomatoes, salsa, and broth, and bring to a boil.
4. Now, reduce the heat to low and simmer for about 15–20 minutes.
5. Stir in the corn and simmer for about 5–10 minutes.
6. Season with salt and black pepper and remove from the heat.
7. Serve hot with the topping of cilantro.

Nutritional Values
- Calories 279
- Total Fat 5.1 g
- Saturated Fat 0.4 g
- Cholesterol 0 mg
- Sodium 308 mg
- Total Carbs 49.3 g
- Fiber 12.6 g
- Sugar 8.8 g
- Protein 14 g

Chili Corn Cane

Preparation time: 15 minutes
Cooking time: 1 hour 10 minutes
Total time: 1 hour 225 minutes
Servings: 10

Ingredients
- 2 tablespoons canola oil
- 2 medium yellow onions, chopped
- 1 large green bell pepper, seeded and chopped
- 5 garlic cloves, minced
- 2 tablespoons ground cumin
- 2 tablespoons ground coriander
- 1 teaspoon ground cinnamon
- 1 tablespoon dried basil, crushed
- 1 tablespoon dried oregano, crushed
- ¼ cup canned tomato puree
- 4¼ cups homemade vegetable broth
- 8 cups canned black beans
- 4 cups tomatoes, chopped
- Salt and ground black pepper, to taste
- ½ cup fresh cilantro, chopped

How to Prepare
1. In a large pan, heat oil over medium-high heat and cook the onion for about 8–9 minutes, stirring frequently.
2. Add the bell pepper, garlic, spices, and herbs, and sauté for about 1 minute.
3. Add the tomato puree, broth, black beans, and tomatoes, and bring to a boil.
4. Now, reduce the heat to low and simmer, covered for about 1 hour.
5. Season with salt and black pepper and remove from the heat.
6. Serve hot with the garnishing of cilantro.

Nutritional Values
- Calories 258
- Total Fat 5.5 g
- Saturated Fat 0.4 g
- Cholesterol 0 mg
- Sodium 373 mg
- Total Carbs 37 g
- Fiber 11.6 g
- Sugar 4.1 g
- Protein 14.9 g

Beans & Quinoa with Veggies

Preparation time: 15 minutes
Cooking time: 30 minutes
Total time: 45 minutes
Servings: 4

Ingredients
- 2 cups water
- 1 cup dry quinoa
- 2 tablespoons coconut oil
- 1 medium white onion, chopped
- 4 garlic cloves, chopped finely
- 2 tablespoons curry powder
- ½ teaspoon ground turmeric
- ½ teaspoon cayenne pepper
- Salt, to taste
- 2 cups green beans, trimmed and chopped
- 2 cups green peas, shelled
- 1 red bell pepper, seeded and chopped
- 2 cups frozen corn, thawed
- 2 tablespoons fresh lime juice

How to Prepare
1. In a pan, add the water and bring to a boil over high heat.
2. Add the quinoa and stir to combine.
3. Reduce the heat to low and simmer for about 10–15 minutes, or until all the liquid is absorbed.
4. In a large cast-iron skillet, melt the coconut oil over medium heat and sauté the onion, garlic, curry powder, turmeric, and salt for about 4–5 minutes.
5. Add the vegetables and cook for about 4–5 minutes.
6. Stir in the quinoa and beans and cook for about 2–3 minutes.
7. Drizzle with the lime juice and serve hot.

Nutritional Values
- Calories 395
- Total Fat 11.3 g
- Saturated Fat 6.5 g
- Cholesterol 0 mg
- Sodium 67 mg
- Total Carbs 64.2 mg
- Fiber 12.9 g
- Sugar 10.2 g
- Protein 14.7 g

Lentil Curry

Preparation time: 15 minutes
Cooking time: 1½ hours
Total time: 1¾ hours
Servings: 8

Ingredients

- 8 cups water
- ½ teaspoon ground turmeric
- 1 cup brown lentils
- 1 cup red lentils
- 1 tablespoon vegetable oil
- 1 large white onion, chopped
- 3 carrots, peeled and chopped
- 3 cups pumpkin, peeled, seeded, and cubed into 1-inch size
- 1 granny smith apple, cored and chopped
- 2 cups fresh spinach, chopped
- Salt and ground black pepper, to taste
- 3 garlic cloves, minced
- 2 tomatoes, seeded and chopped
- 1½ tablespoons curry powder
- ¼ teaspoon ground cloves
- 2 teaspoons ground cumin

How to Prepare

1. In a large pan, add the water, turmeric, and lentils over high heat and bring to a boil.
2. Now, reduce the heat to medium-low and simmer, covered for about 30 minutes.
3. Drain the lentils, reserving 2½ cups of the cooking liquid.
4. Meanwhile, in another large pan, heat the oil over medium heat and sauté the onion for about 2–3 minutes.
5. Add in the garlic and sauté for about 1 minute.
6. Add the tomatoes and cook for about 5 minutes.
7. Stir in the curry powder and spices and cook for about 1 minute.
8. Add the carrots, potatoes, pumpkin, cooked lentils, and reserved cooking liquid and bring to a gentle boil.
9. Reduce the heat to medium-low and simmer, covered for about 40–45 minutes or until desired doneness of the vegetables.
10. Stir in the apple and spinach and simmer for about 15 minutes.
11. Stir in the salt and black pepper and remove from the heat.
12. Serve hot.

Nutritional Values

- Calories 263
- Total Fat 2.9 g
- Saturated Fat 0.6 g
- Cholesterol 0 mg
- Sodium 53 mg
- Total Carbs 47 g
- Fiber 20 g
- Sugar 9.7 g
- Protein 14.7 g

Nut Roast Dinner

Preparation time: 15 minutes
Cooking time: 1½ hours
Total time: 1¾ hours
Servings: 6

Ingredients

- ½ tablespoon olive oil
- 2 yellow onions, chopped
- ½ cup celery stalk, chopped
- 1 teaspoon dried rosemary, crushed
- 1 teaspoon dried basil, crushed
- ¾ cup pecans, chopped
- ¾ cup walnuts, chopped
- 3 cups whole-wheat breadcrumbs
- 2½ cups unsweetened soymilk
- Salt and ground black pepper, to taste

How to Prepare

1. Preheat the oven to 350ºF. Lightly grease a loaf pan.
2. In a large bowl, add all the ingredients and mix until well combined.
3. Transfer the mixture into prepared loaf pan.
4. Bake for about 60–90 minutes, or until top become golden-brown.
5. Remove from the oven and place the loaf pan onto a wire rack for about 10 minutes.
6. Carefully, invert the loaf onto a platter.
7. Cut into desired-sized slices and serve.

Nutritional Values

- Calories 429
- Total Fat 24.6 g
- Saturated Fat 2.1 g
- Cholesterol 0 mg
- Sodium 143 mg
- Total Carbs 42 g
- Fiber 8.4 g
- Sugar 7.5 g
- Protein 15.3 g

Rice & Lentil Casserole

Preparation time: 20 minutes
Cooking time: 1 hour
Total time: 1 hour 20 minutes
Servings: 6

Ingredients

- 2½ cups water, divided
- 1 cup red lentils
- ½ cup wild rice
- 1 teaspoon olive oil
- 1 small onion, chopped
- 3 garlic cloves, minced
- 1/3 cup zucchini, chopped
- 1/3 cup carrot, peeled and chopped
- 1/3 cup celery stalk, chopped
- 1 fresh tomato, chopped
- 8 ounces tomato sauce
- 1 teaspoon ground cumin
- 1 teaspoon dried oregano, crushed
- 1 teaspoon dried basil, crushed
- Salt and ground black pepper, to taste

How to Prepare

1. In a pan, add 1 cup of the water and rice over medium-high heat and bring to a rolling boil.
2. Now, lower the heat to low and simmer, covered for about 20 minutes.
3. Meanwhile, in another pan, add the remaining water and lentils over medium heat and bring to a rolling boil.
4. Now, lower the heat to low and simmer, covered for about 15 minutes.
5. Transfer the cooked rice and lentils into a casserole dish and set aside.
6. Preheat your oven to 350ºF.
7. Heat the oil in a large skillet over medium heat and sauté the onion and garlic for about 4–5 minutes.
8. Add the zucchini, carrot, celery, tomato, and tomato paste, and cook for about 4–5 minutes.
9. Stir in the cumin, herbs, salt, and black pepper, and remove from the heat.
10. Transfer the vegetable mixture into the casserole dish with rice and lentils and stir to combine.
11. Bake for about 30 minutes.
12. Remove from the heat and set aside for about 5 minutes.
13. Cut into equal-sized 6 pieces and serve.

Nutritional Values

- Calories 192
- Total Fat 1.5 g
- Saturated Fat 0.2 g
- Cholesterol 0 mg
- Sodium 239 mg
- Total Carbs 34.5 g
- Fiber 12 g
- Sugar 3.9 g
- Protein 11.3 g

Pasta & Veggie Casserole

Preparation time: 15 minutes
Cooking time: 1 hour 10 minutes
Total time: 1 hour 25 minutes
Servings: 6

Ingredients

Sauce
- 1 cup sunflower seeds, shelled, soaked for 30 minutes, drained and rinsed
- ¼ cup low-sodium soy sauce
- 1½ cups water
- Pinch of ground black pepper

Casserole
- 1 (14-ounce) package whole-wheat fusilli pasta
- 2 tablespoons extra-virgin olive oil
- 3 cups Brussels sprouts, trimmed and quartered
- Salt and ground black pepper, to taste
- 1 cup water
- 1 (14-ounce) package frozen spinach, thawed

How to Prepare

1. Preheat the oven to 400ºF. Grease large baking dish.
2. For sauce: in a blender, add all the ingredients and pulse until smooth.
3. Transfer the sauce into a bowl and set aside.
4. In a pan of the boiling water, add the pasta and cook for about 8–10 minutes.
5. Drain the pasta well and set aside.
6. Meanwhile, in a large skillet, heat the oil over medium heat and cook the Brussels sprouts and black pepper for about 3–4 minutes.
7. Add the water and cook for about 8–10 minutes.
8. Stir in the spinach and cook for about 1 minute.
9. Stir in the sauce and cook for about 1 minute.
10. Stir in the cooked pasta and remove from the heat.
11. Transfer the pasta mixture into prepared baking dish.
12. Bake for about 35 minutes.
13. Remove from the oven and set aside for about 5 minutes before serving.

Nutritional Values
- Calories 371
- Total Fat 10.8 g
- Saturated Fat 1.1 g
- Cholesterol 0 mg
- Sodium 702 mg
- Total Carbs 57.9 g
- Fiber 9.7 g
- Sugar 3.9 g

VEGETABLE RECIPES

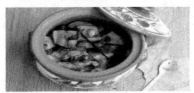

Dried Fruit Squash

Preparation time: 15 minutes
Cooking time: 40 minutes
Total time: 55 minutes
Servings: 4

Ingredients
- ¼ cup water
- 1 medium butternut squash, halved and seeded
- ½ tablespoon olive oil
- ½ tablespoon balsamic vinegar
- Salt and ground black pepper, to taste
- 4 large dates, pitted and chopped
- 4 fresh figs, chopped
- 3 tablespoons pistachios, chopped
- 2 tablespoons pumpkin seeds

How to Prepare
1. Preheat the oven to 375ºF.
2. Place the water in the bottom of a baking dish.
3. Arrange the squash halves in a large baking dish, hollow-side up, and drizzle with oil and vinegar.
4. Sprinkle with salt and black pepper.
5. Spread the dates, figs, and pistachios on top.
6. Bake for about 40 minutes, or until squash becomes tender.
7. Serve hot with the garnishing of pumpkin seeds.

Nutritional Values
- Calories 227
- Total Fat 5.5 g
- Saturated Fat 0.8 g
- Cholesterol 0 mg
- Sodium 66 mg
- Total Carbs 46.4 g
- Fiber 7.5 g
- Sugar 19.6 g
- Protein 5 g

Banana Curry

Preparation time: 15 minutes
Cooking time: 15 minutes
Total time: 30 minutes
Servings: 3

Ingredients
- 2 tablespoons olive oil
- 2 yellow onions, chopped
- 8 garlic cloves, minced
- 2 tablespoons curry powder
- 1 tablespoon ground ginger
- 1 tablespoon ground cumin
- 1 teaspoon ground turmeric
- 1 teaspoon ground cinnamon
- 1 teaspoon red chili powder
- Salt and ground black pepper, to taste
- 2/3 cup soy yogurt
- 1 cup tomato puree
- 2 bananas, peeled and sliced
- 3 tomatoes, chopped finely
- ¼ cup unsweetened coconut flakes

How to Prepare
1. In a large pan, heat the oil over medium heat and sauté onion for about 4–5 minutes.
2. Add the garlic, curry powder, and spices, and sauté for about 1 minute.
3. Add the soy yogurt and tomato sauce and bring to a gentle boil.
4. Stir in the bananas and simmer for about 3 minutes.
5. Stir in the tomatoes and simmer for about 1–2 minutes.
6. Stir in the coconut flakes and immediately remove from the heat.
7. Serve hot.

Nutritional Values
- Calories 382
- Total Fat 18.2 g
- Saturated Fat 6.6 g
- Cholesterol 0 mg
- Sodium 108 mg
- Total Carbs 53.4 g
- Fiber 11.3 g
- Sugar 24.8 g
- Protein 9 g

Mushroom Curry

Preparation time: 15 minutes
Cooking time: 20 minutes
Total time: 35 minutes
Servings: 3

Ingredients
- 2 cups tomatoes, chopped
- 1 green chili, chopped
- 1 teaspoon fresh ginger, chopped
- ¼ cup cashews
- 2 tablespoons canola oil
- ½ teaspoon cumin seeds
- ¼ teaspoon ground coriander
- ¼ teaspoon ground turmeric
- ¼ teaspoon red chili powder
- 1½ cups fresh shiitake mushrooms, sliced
- 1½ cups fresh button mushrooms, sliced
- 1 cup frozen corn kernels
- 1¼ cups water
- ¼ cup unsweetened coconut milk
- Salt and ground black pepper, to taste

How to Prepare
1. In a food processor, add the tomatoes, green chili, ginger, and cashews, and pulse until a smooth paste forms.
2. In a pan, heat the oil over medium heat and sauté the cumin seeds for about 1 minute.
3. Add the spices and sauté for about 1 minute.
4. Add the tomato paste and cook for about 5 minutes.
5. Stir in the mushrooms, corn, water, and coconut milk, and bring to a boil.
6. Cook for about 10–12 minutes, stirring occasionally.
7. Season with salt and black pepper and remove from the heat.
8. Serve hot.

Nutritional Values
- Calories 311
- Total Fat 20.4 g
- Saturated Fat 6.1 g
- Cholesterol 0 mg
- Sodium 244 mg
- Total Carbs 32g
- Fiber 5.6 g
- Sugar 9 g
- Protein 8 g

3-Veggie Combo

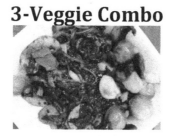

Preparation time: 15 minutes
Cooking time: 25 minutes
Total time: 40 minutes
Servings: 4

Ingredients
- 1 tablespoon olive oil
- 1 small yellow onion, chopped
- 1 teaspoon fresh thyme, chopped
- 1 garlic clove, minced
- 8 ounces fresh button mushroom, sliced
- 1 pound Brussels sprouts
- 3 cups fresh spinach
- 4 tablespoons walnuts
- Salt and ground black pepper, to taste

How to Prepare
1. In a large skillet, heat the oil over medium heat and sauté the onion for about 3–4 minutes.
2. Add the thyme and garlic and sauté for about 1 minute.
3. Add the mushrooms and cook for about 15 minutes, or until caramelized.
4. Add the Brussels sprouts and cook for about 2–3 minutes.
5. Stir in the spinach and cook for about 3–4 minutes.
6. Stir in the walnuts, salt, and black pepper, and remove from the heat.
7. Serve hot.

Nutritional Values
- Calories 153
- Total Fat 8.8 g
- Saturated Fat 0.9 g
- Cholesterol 0 mg
- Sodium 94 mg
- Total Carbs 15.8 g
- Fiber 6.3 g
- Sugar 4.4 g
- Protein 8.5 g

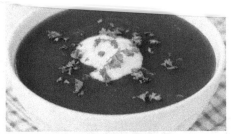

Beet Soup

Preparation time: 10 minutes
Cooking time: 5 minutes
Total time: 15 minutes
Servings: 2

Ingredients
- 2 cups coconut yogurt
- 4 teaspoons fresh lemon juice
- 2 cups beets, trimmed, peeled, and chopped
- 2 tablespoons fresh dill
- Salt, to taste
- 1 tablespoon pumpkin seeds
- 2 tablespoons coconut cream
- 1 tablespoon fresh chives, minced

How to Prepare
1. In a high-speed blender, add all ingredients and pulse until smooth.
2. Transfer the soup into a pan over medium heat and cook for about 3–5 minutes or until heated through.
3. Serve immediately with the garnishing of chives and coconut cream.

Nutritional Values
- Calories 230
- Total Fat 8 g
- Saturated Fat 5.8 g
- Cholesterol 0 mg
- Sodium 218 mg
- Total Carbs 33.5 g
- Fiber 4.2 g
- Sugar 27.5 g
- Protein 8 g

Veggie Stew

Preparation time: 15 minutes
Cooking time: 30 minutes
Total time: 45 minutes
Servings: 3

Ingredients
- 2 tablespoons olive oil
- 1 large onion, chopped
- 2 garlic cloves, minced
- ¼ teaspoon fresh ginger, grated finely
- 1 teaspoon ground cumin
- 1 teaspoon cayenne pepper
- Salt and ground black pepper, to taste
- 2 cups homemade vegetable broth
- 1½ cups small broccoli florets
- 1½ cups small cauliflower florets
- 1 tablespoon fresh lemon juice
- 1 cup cashews
- 1 teaspoon fresh lemon zest, grated finely

How to Prepare
1. In a large soup pan, heat oil over medium heat and sauté the onion for about 3–4 minutes.
2. Add the garlic, ginger, and spices and sauté for about 1 minute.
3. Add 1 cup of the broth and bring to a boil.
4. Add the vegetables and again bring to a boil.
5. Cover the soup pan and cook for about 15–20 minutes, stirring occasionally.
6. Stir in the lemon juice and remove from the heat.
7. Serve hot with the topping of cashews and lemon zest.

Nutritional Values
- Calories 425
- Total Fat 32 g
- Saturated Fat 5.9 g
- Cholesterol 0 mg
- Sodium 601 mg
- Total Carbs 27.6 g
- Fiber 5.2 g
- Sugar 7.1 g
- Protein 13.4 g

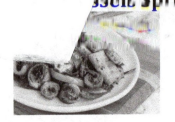

Preparation time: 15 minutes
Cooking time: 15 minutes
Total time: 30 minutes
Servings: 3

Ingredients
- 1½ tablespoons olive oil, divided
- 8 ounces extra-firm tofu, drained, pressed, and cut into slices
- 2 garlic cloves, chopped
- 1/3 cup pecans, toasted, and chopped
- 1 tablespoon unsweetened applesauce
- ¼ cup fresh cilantro, chopped
- ½ pound Brussels sprouts, trimmed and cut into wide ribbons
- ¾ pound mixed bell peppers, seeded and sliced

How to Prepare
1. In a skillet, heat ½ tablespoon of the oil over medium heat and sauté the tofu and for about 6–7 minutes, or until golden-brown.
2. Add the garlic and pecans and sauté for about 1 minute.
3. Add the applesauce and cook for about 2 minutes.
4. Stir in the cilantro and remove from heat.
5. Transfer tofu into a plate and set aside
6. In the same skillet, heat the remaining oil over medium-high heat and cook the Brussels sprouts and bell peppers for about 5 minutes.
7. Stir in the tofu and remove from the heat.
8. Serve immediately.

Nutritional Values
- Calories 238
- Total Fat 17.8 g
- Saturated Fat 2 g
- Cholesterol 0 mg
- Sodium 26 mg
- Total Carbs 13.6 g
- Fiber 4.8 g
- Sugar 4.5 g
- Protein 11.8 g

Tofu with Peas

Preparation time: 15 minutes
Cooking time: 20 minutes
Total time: 35 minutes
Servings: 5

Ingredients
- 1 tablespoon chili-garlic sauce
- 3 tablespoons low-sodium soy sauce
- 2 tablespoons canola oil, divided
- 1 (16-ounce) package extra-firm tofu, drained, pressed, and cubed
- 1 cup yellow onion, chopped
- 1 tablespoon fresh ginger, minced
- 2 garlic cloves, minced
- 2 large tomatoes, chopped finely
- 5 cups frozen peas, thawed
- 1 teaspoon white sesame seeds

How to Prepare
1. For sauce: in a bowl, add the chili-garlic sauce and soy sauce and mix until well combined.
2. In a large skillet, heat 1 tablespoon of oil over medium-high heat and cook the tofu for about 4–5 minutes or until browned completely, stirring occasionally.
3. Transfer the tofu into a bowl.
4. In the same skillet, heat the remaining oil over medium heat and sauté the onion for about 3–4 minutes.
5. Add the ginger and garlic and sauté for about 1 minute.
6. Add the tomatoes and cook for about 4–5 minutes, crushing with the back of spoon.
7. Stir in all three peas and cook for about 2–3 minutes.
8. Stir in the sauce mixture and tofu and cook for about 1–2 minutes.
9. Serve hot with the garnishing of sesame seeds.

Nutritional Values
- Calories 291
- Total Fat 11.9 g
- Saturated Fat 1.1 g
- Cholesterol 0 mg
- Sodium 732 mg
- Total Carbs 31.6 g
- Fiber 10.8 g
- Sugar 11.5 g
- Protein 19 g

Carrot Soup with Tempeh

Preparation time: 15 minutes
Cooking time: 45 minutes
Total time: 1 hour
Servings: 6

Ingredients
- ¼ cup olive oil, divided
- 1 large yellow onion, chopped
- Salt, to taste
- 2 pounds carrots, peeled, and cut into ½-inch rounds
- 2 tablespoons fresh dill, chopped
- 4½ cups homemade vegetable broth
- 12 ounces tempeh, cut into ½-inch cubes
- ¼ cup tomato paste
- 1 teaspoon fresh lemon juice

How to Prepare
1. In a large soup pan, heat 2 tablespoons of the oil over medium heat and cook the onion with salt for about 6–8 minutes, stirring frequently.
2. Add the carrots and stir to combine.
3. Lower the heat to low and cook, covered for about 5 minutes, stirring frequently.
4. Add in the broth and bring to a boil over high heat.
5. Lower the heat to a low and simmer, covered for about 30 minutes.
6. Meanwhile, in a skillet, heat the remaining oil over medium-high heat and cook the tempeh for about 3–5 minutes.
7. Stir in the dill and cook for about 1 minute.
8. Remove from the heat.
9. Remove the pan of soup from heat and stir in tomato paste and lemon juice.
10. With an immersion blender, blend the soup until smooth and creamy.
11. Serve the soup hot with the topping of tempeh.

Nutritional Values
- Calories 294
- Total Fat 15.7 g
- Saturated Fat 2.8 g
- Cholesterol 0 mg
- Sodium 723 mg
- Total Carbs 25.9 g
- Fiber 4.9 g
- Sugar 10.4 g
- Protein 16.4 g

Tempeh with Bell Peppers

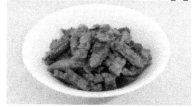

Preparation time: 15 minutes
Cooking time: 15 minutes
Total time: 30 minutes
Servings: 3

Ingredients
- 2 tablespoons balsamic vinegar
- 2 tablespoons low-sodium soy sauce
- 2 tablespoons tomato sauce
- 1 teaspoon maple syrup
- ½ teaspoon garlic powder
- 1/8 teaspoon red pepper flakes, crushed
- 1 tablespoon vegetable oil
- 8 ounces tempeh, cut into cubes
- 1 medium onion, chopped
- 2 large green bell peppers, seeded and chopped

How to Prepare
1. In a small bowl, add the vinegar, soy sauce, tomato sauce, maple syrup, garlic powder, and red pepper flakes and beat until well combined. Set aside.
2. Heat 1 tablespoon of oil in a large skillet over medium heat and cook the tempeh about 2–3 minutes per side.
3. Add the onion and bell peppers and heat for about 2–3 minutes.
4. Stir in the sauce mixture and cook for about 3–5 minutes, stirring frequently.
5. Serve hot.

Nutritional Values
- Calories 241
- Total Fat 13 g
- Saturated Fat 2.6 g
- Cholesterol 0 mg
- Sodium 65 mg
- Total Carbs 19.7 g
- Fiber 2.1 g
- Sugar 8.1 g
- Protein 16.1 g

QUICK ENERGY & RECOVERY SNACKS RECIPES

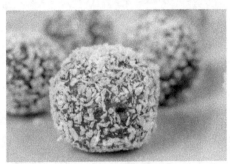

Date & Seed Bites

Preparation time: 15 minutes
Total time: 15 minutes
Servings: 10

Ingredients
- 1 cup cashew butter
- 6 Medjool dates, pitted
- 2/3 cup hemp seeds
- ¼ cup chia seeds
- ¼ cup unsweetened vegan protein powder
- ¾ cup unsweetened coconut, shredded

How to Prepare
1. In a food processor, place all the ingredients and pulse until well combined.
2. With your hands, make equal-sized balls from mixture.
3. In a shallow dish, place the coconut.
4. Roll the balls in the coconut evenly.
5. Refrigerate the balls till serving.
6. Arrange the balls onto a parchment paper-lined baking sheet in a single layer.
7. Refrigerate to set for about 30 minutes before serving.

Nutritional Values:
- Calories 350
- Total Fat 25.3 g
- Saturated Fat 9.2 g
- Cholesterol 0 mg
- Sodium 188 mg
- Total Carbs 24.1 g
- Fiber 4.5 g
- Sugar 11.4 g
- Protein 12.4 g

Chocolatey Oat Bites

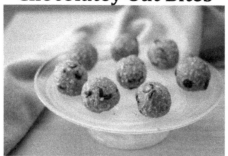

Preparation time: 15 minutes
Total time: 15 minutes
Servings: 6
Ingredients
- 2/3 cup creamy peanut butter
- 1 cup old-fashioned oats
- ½ cups unsweetened vegan chocolate chips
- ½ cups ground flaxseeds
- 2 tablespoons maple syrup

How to Prepare
1. In a bowl, place all the ingredients and mix until well combined.
2. Refrigerate for about 20–30 minutes.
3. With your hands, make equal-sized balls from mixture.
4. Arrange the balls onto a parchment paper-lined baking sheet in a single layer.
5. Refrigerate to set for about 15 minutes before serving.

Nutritional Values
- Calories 473
- Total Fat 29.8 g
- Saturated Fat 10.5 g
- Cholesterol 0 mg
- Sodium 141 mg
- Total Carbs 36 g
- Fiber 9.5 g
- Sugar 7.5 g
- Protein 14.9 g

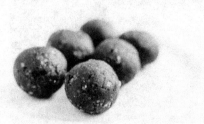

Brownie Bites

Preparation time: 15 minutes
Total time: 15 minutes
Servings: 8

Ingredients
- ¾ cup blanched almond flour
- ¾ cup cacao powder
- 2 tablespoons ground flaxseed
- ½ cup unsweetened vegan mini chocolate chips
- ¾ cup creamy almond butter, melted
- ¼ cup pure maple syrup
- 1 teaspoon pure vanilla extract

How to Prepare
1. In a large bowl, mix together the almond flour, cocoa powder, flaxseed, and chocolate chips.
2. Add the almond butter, maple syrup, and vanilla extract, and gently stir to combine.
3. Using a sturdy spatula, stir and fold together until well incorporated.
4. With your hands, make equal-sized balls from mixture.
5. Arrange the balls onto a parchment paper-lined baking sheet in a single layer.
6. Refrigerate to set for about 15 minutes before serving.

Nutritional Values
- Calories 360
- Total Fat 27.4 g
- Saturated Fat 8 g
- Cholesterol 0 mg
- Sodium 61 mg
- Total Carbs 23.1 g
- Fiber 8.5 g
- Sugar 8.4 g
- Protein 10.7 g

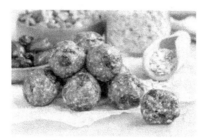

Fruity Bites

Preparation time: 15 minutes
Total time: 15 minutes
Servings: 6

Ingredients
- 1 ripe banana, peeled
- ¼ cup maple syrup
- ¼ cup sunflower seed butter, melted
- 1½ cups quick oats
- ¾ cup rolled oats
- 1/3 cup unsweetened vegan protein powder
- 2 teaspoons ground flaxseed
- 1 teaspoon vanilla extract
- 1/3 cup dried unsweetened cranberries

How to Prepare
1. In a large bowl, add the banana and with a fork, mash it.
2. Add the maple syrup and sunflower seed butter and mix until smooth.
3. Add the oats, protein powder, flaxseed, and vanilla extract and mix until well combined.
4. Gently, fold in the cranberries.
5. With your hands, make equal-sized balls from mixture.
6. Arrange the balls onto a parchment paper-lined baking sheet in a single layer.
7. Refrigerate to set for about 15 minutes before serving.

Nutritional Values
- Calories 269
- Total Fat 7.8 g
- Saturated Fat 0.9 g
- Cholesterol 0 mg
- Sodium 69 mg
- Total Carbs 38 g
- Fiber 5 g
- Sugar 11.2 g
- Protein 12.9 g

Energy Bars

Preparation time: 15 minutes
Total time: 15 minutes
Servings: 8

Ingredients
- 1½ cups rolled oats
- ½ cup almonds, chopped roughly
- ½ cup cashews, chopped roughly
- ½ cup mini unsweetened vegan chocolate chips
- 1/3 cup pumpkin seeds
- ¼ cup sesame seeds
- ¼ cup sunflower seeds
- ¼ cup flaxseed meal
- 2 tablespoons chia seeds
- 1 teaspoon ground cinnamon
- ½ cup maple syrup
- 1 cup almond butter, softened

How to Prepare
1. Line an 8x8-inch baking dish with a large lightly greased parchment paper.
2. In a large bowl, add oats, nuts, chocolate chips, seeds, and cinnamon, and mix well.
3. Add in the maple syrup and stir to combine.
4. Add the almond butter and mix until well combined.
5. Place oat mixture into prepared baking dish evenly and with the back of a spatula, smooth the top surface, by pressing in the bottom.
6. Refrigerate for about 6–8 hours, or until set completely.
7. Remove from refrigerator and with a sharp knife, cut into desired sized bars.

Nutritional Values
- Calories 397
- Total Fat 24.5 g
- Saturated Fat 7.4 g
- Cholesterol 0 mg
- Sodium 12 mg
- Total Carbs 36.4 g
- Fiber 7.4 g
- Sugar 12.8 g
- Protein 10.7 g

DRINKS & DESSERT RECIPES

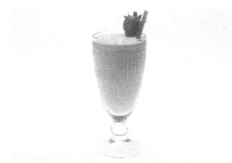

Strawberry Shake

Preparation time: 10 minutes
Total time: 10 minutes
Servings: 2

Ingredients
- 1½ cups fresh strawberries, hulled
- 1 large frozen banana, peeled
- 2 scoops unsweetened vegan vanilla protein powder
- 2 tablespoons hemp seeds
- 2 cups unsweetened hemp milk

How to Prepare
1. In a high-speed blender, place all the ingredients and pulse until creamy.
2. Pour into two glasses and serve immediately.

Nutritional Values
- Calories 325
- Total Fat 13 g
- Saturated Fat 0.8 g
- Cholesterol 0 mg
- Sodium 391 mg
- Total Carbs 23.3 g
- Fiber 3.9 g
- Sugar 12.5 g
- Protein 31.2 g

Chocolatey Banana Shake

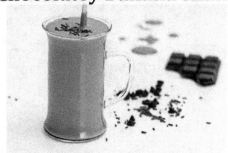

Preparation time: 10 minutes
Total time: 10 minutes
Servings: 2

Ingredients
- 2 medium frozen bananas, peeled
- 4 dates, pitted
- 4 tablespoons peanut butter
- 4 tablespoons rolled oats
- 2 tablespoons cacao powder
- 2 tablespoons chia seeds
- 2 cups unsweetened soymilk

How to Prepare
1. Place all the ingredients in a high-speed blender and pulse until creamy.
2. Pour into two glasses and serve immediately.

Nutritional Values
- Calories 583
- Total Fat 25.2 g
- Saturated Fat 4.8 g
- Cholesterol 0 mg
- Sodium 200 mg
- Total Carbs 75 g
- Fiber 15.3 g
- Sugar 37.8 g
- Protein 23.1 g

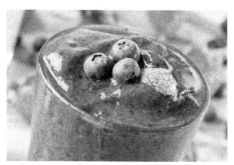

Fruity Tofu Smoothie

Preparation time: 10 minutes
Total time: 10 minutes
Servings: 2

Ingredients
- 12 ounces silken tofu, pressed and drained
- 2 medium bananas, peeled
- 1½ cups fresh blueberries
- 1 tablespoon maple syrup
- 1½ cups unsweetened soymilk
- ¼ cup ice cubes

How to Prepare
1. Place all the ingredients in a high-speed blender and pulse until creamy.
2. Pour into two glasses and serve immediately.

Nutritional Values
- Calories 398
- Total Fat 8.6 g
- Saturated Fat 1.2 g
- Cholesterol 0 mg
- Sodium 58 mg
- Total Carbs 65 g
- Fiber 7 g
- Sugar 50.7 g
- Protein 19.9 g

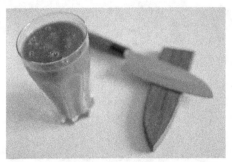

Green Fruity Smoothie

Preparation time: 10 minutes
Total time: 10 minutes
Servings: 2

Ingredients
- 1 cup frozen mango, peeled, pitted, and chopped
- 1 large frozen banana, peeled
- 2 cups fresh baby spinach
- 1 scoop unsweetened vegan vanilla protein powder
- ¼ cup pumpkin seeds
- 2 tablespoons hemp hearts
- 1½ cups unsweetened almond milk

How to Prepare
1. In a high-speed blender, place all the ingredients and pulse until creamy.
2. Pour into two glasses and serve immediately.

Nutritional Values
- Calories 355
- Total Fat 16.1 g
- Saturated Fat 2.4 g
- Cholesterol 0 mg
- Sodium 295 mg
- Total Carbs 34.6 g
- Fiber 6.2 g
- Sugar 19.9 g
- Protein 23.4 g

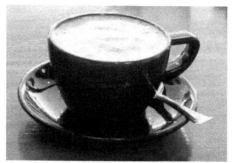

Protein Latte

Preparation time: 10 minutes
Total time: 10 minutes
Servings: 2

Ingredients
- 2 cups hot brewed coffee
- 1¼ cups coconut milk
- 2 teaspoons coconut oil
- 2 scoops unsweetened vegan vanilla protein powder

How to Prepare
1. Place all the ingredients in a high-speed blender and pulse until creamy.
2. Pour into two serving mugs and serve immediately.

Nutritional Values
- Calories 503
- Total Fat 41.4 g
- Saturated Fat 35.6 g
- Cholesterol 0 mg
- Sodium 291 mg
- Total Carbs 8.3 g
- Fiber 3.3 g
- Sugar 5 g
- Protein 29.1 g

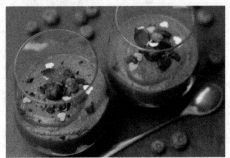

Chocolatey Bean Mousse

Preparation time: 10 minutes
Total time: 10 minutes
Servings: 3

Ingredients
- ½ cup unsweetened almond milk
- 1 cup cooked black beans
- 4 Medjool dates, pitted and chopped
- ½ cup walnuts, chopped
- 2 tablespoons cacao powder
- 1 teaspoon vanilla extract
- 3 tablespoons fresh blueberries
- 1 teaspoon fresh mint leaves

How to Prepare
1. In a food processor, add all ingredients and pulse until smooth and creamy.
2. Transfer the mousse into serving bowls and refrigerate to chill before serving.
3. Garnish with blueberries and mint leaves and serve.

Nutritional Values
- Calories 465
- Total Fat 14.5 g
- Saturated Fat 1.4 g
- Cholesterol 0 mg
- Sodium 34 mg
- Total Carbs 69.9 g
- Fiber 15 g
- Sugar 23.3 g
- Protein 21.1 g

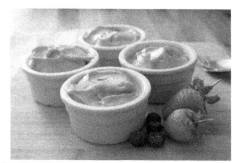

Tofu & Strawberry Mousse

Preparation time: 10 minutes
Total time: 10 minutes
Servings: 4

Ingredients
- 2 cups fresh strawberries, hulled and sliced
- 2 cups firm tofu, pressed and drained
- 3 tablespoons maple syrup
- 4 tablespoons walnuts, chopped

How to Prepare
1. In a blender, add the strawberries and pulse until just pureed.
2. Add the tofu and maple syrup and pulse until smooth.
3. Transfer the mousse into serving bowls and refrigerate to chill before serving.
4. Garnish with walnuts and serve.

Nutritional Values
- Calories 199
- Total Fat 10.1 g
- Saturated Fat 1.4 g
- Cholesterol 0 mg
- Sodium 17 mg
- Total Carbs 18.5 g
- Fiber 3.1 g
- Sugar 13.3 g
- Protein 12.7 g

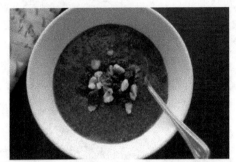

Tofu & Chia Seed Pudding

Preparation time: 15 minutes
Total time: 15 minutes
Servings: 4

Ingredients
- 1 pound silken tofu, pressed and drained
- ¼ cup banana, peeled
- 3 tablespoons cacao powder
- 1 teaspoon vanilla extract
- 3 tablespoons chia seeds
- ¼ cup walnuts, chopped
- ¼ cup black raisins

How to Prepare
1. In a food processor, add tofu, banana, cocoa powder, and vanilla, and pulse till smooth and creamy.
2. Transfer into a large serving bowl and stir in chia seeds till well mixed.
3. Now, place the pudding in serving bowls evenly.
4. With plastic wraps, cover the bowls. Refrigerate to chill before serving.
5. Garnish with raspberries and serve.

Nutritional Values
- Calories 188
- Total Fat 10.4 g
- Saturated Fat 1.4 g
- Cholesterol 0 mg
- Sodium 42 mg
- Total Carbs 17.1 g
- Fiber 4.2 g
- Sugar 8.2 g
- Protein 12 g

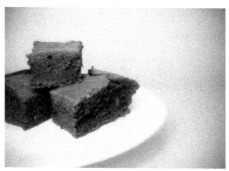

Banana Brownies

Preparation time: 15 minutes
Cooking time: 20 minutes
Total time: 35 minutes
Servings: 8

Ingredients
- 6 bananas
- 2 scoops unsweetened vegan vanilla protein powder
- 1 cup creamy peanut butter
- ½ cup cacao powder

How to Prepare
1. Preheat the oven the 350ºF. Line a square baking dish with greased parchment paper.
2. In a food processor, add all the ingredients and pulse until smooth.
3. Transfer the mixture into the prepared baking dish evenly and with the back of a spatula, smooth the top surface.
4. Bake for about 18–20 minutes.
5. Remove from oven and place onto a wire rack to cool completely.
6. With a sharp knife, cut into equal-sized brownies and serve.

Nutritional Values
- Calories 310
- Total Fat 17.8 g
- Saturated Fat 4.2 g
- Cholesterol 0 mg
- Sodium 215 mg
- Total Carbs 29.1 g
- Fiber 5.7 g
- Sugar 13.7 g
- Protein 16.4 g

Brown Rice Pudding

Preparation time: 15 minutes
Cooking time: 1¼ hours
Total time: 1¾ hours
Servings: 2

Ingredients
- ½ cup brown basmati rice, soaked for 15 minutes and drained
- 1½ cups water
- 2½ cups unsweetened almond milk
- 4 tablespoons cashews
- 2–3 tablespoons maple syrup
- 1/8 teaspoon ground cardamom
- Pinch of salt
- 3 tablespoons golden raisins
- 2 tablespoons cashews
- 2 tablespoons almonds

How to Prepare
1. In a pan, add the rice and water over medium-high heat and bring to a boil.
2. Lower the heat to medium and cook for about 30 minutes.
3. Meanwhile, in a blender, add the almond milk and cashews and pulse until smooth.
4. In the pan of rice, slowly add the milk mixture stirring continuously.
5. Sir in the maple syrup, cardamom, and salt, and cook for about 15–20 minutes, stirring occasionally.
6. Stir in the raisins and cook for about 15–20 minutes, stirring occasionally.
7. Remove from the heat and set aside to cool slightly.
8. Serve warm with the garnishing of banana slices and pistachios.

Nutritional Values
- Calories 498
- Total Fat 20.7 g
- Saturated Fat 3.2 g
- Cholesterol 0 mg
- Sodium 317 mg
- Total Carbs 72.7 g
- Fiber 4.9 g
- Sugar 21.5 g
- Protein 10.5 g

SAUCES RECIPES

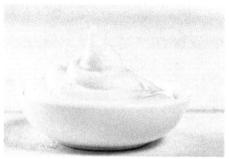

Tofu Mayonnaise

Preparation time: 15 minutes
Total time: 15 minutes
Servings: 6

Ingredients
- ½ pound silken tofu, pressed
- ½ of garlic clove, chopped finely
- 2 tablespoons fresh lemon juice
- 2 tablespoons Dijon mustard
- Freshly ground black pepper, to taste
- ½ cup canola oil

How to Prepare
1. In a blender, add tofu, garlic, lemon juice, mustard, and black pepper, and pulse until smooth.
2. While the motor is running, slowly add oil and pulse on low speed until well combined.
3. Transfer into a bowl and serve.

Nutritional Values
- Calories 142
- Total Fat 14.6 g
- Saturated Fat 1.2 g
- Cholesterol 0 mg
- Sodium 55 mg
- Total Carbs 1 g
- Fiber 0.2 g
- Sugar 0.5 g
- Protein 2.2 g

Chickpea Hummus

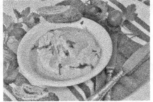

Preparation time: 15 minutes
Total time: 15 minutes
Servings: 6

Ingredients
- ¼ cup tahini, well-stirred
- ¼ cup fresh lemon juice
- 1 small garlic clove, minced
- 3 tablespoons extra-virgin olive oil, divided
- ½ teaspoon ground cumin
- 1 (15-ounce) can chickpeas, rinsed and drained
- 2–3 tablespoons water
- Pinch of paprika

How to Prepare
1. In a food processor, add the tahini and lemon juice and pulse for about 1 minute.
2. Add the garlic, 2 tablespoons of oil, and cumin, and pulse for about 30 seconds.
3. Scrape the sides and bottom of food processor and pulse for about 30 seconds more.
4. Add half of the chickpeas and pulse for about 1 minute.
5. Scrape sides and bottom of the food processor.
6. Add remaining chickpeas and pulse for about 1–2 minutes or, until just smooth.
7. Add water and pulse until smooth.
8. Place the hummus into a serving bowl and drizzle with the remaining oil.
9. Sprinkle with paprika and serve.

Nutritional Values
- Calories 187
- Total Fat 13.4 g
- Saturated Fat 2 g
- Cholesterol 0 mg
- Sodium 132 mg
- Total Carbs 12.9 g
- Fiber 3.1 g
- Sugar 0.6 g
- Protein 6 g

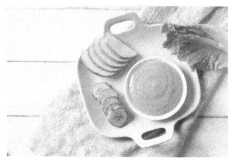

Peanut Butter Sauce

Preparation time: 10 minutes
Total time: 10 minutes
Servings: 3

Ingredients
- ½ cup creamy peanut butter
- 2 tablespoons low-sodium soy sauce
- 1 tablespoon maple syrup
- 2 tablespoons fresh lime juice
- 1 teaspoon chile garlic sauce
- ¼ cup water

How to Prepare
1. In a bowl, place all the ingredients and beat until well combined.
2. Serve immediately.

Nutritional Values
- Calories 274
- Total Fat 21.7 g
- Saturated Fat 4.6 g
- Cholesterol 0 mg
- Sodium 827 mg
- Total Carbs 13.7 g
- Fiber 2.6 g
- Sugar 8.7 g
- Protein 11.4 g

Tomato Sauce

Preparation time: 20 minutes
Cooking time: 4 hours 20 minutes
Total time: 4 hours 40 minutes
Servings: 6

Ingredients
- 10 ripe tomatoes
- 3 tablespoons olive oil
- 2 carrots, peeled and chopped
- 1 green bell pepper, seeded and chopped
- 1 yellow onion, chopped
- 4 garlic cloves, minced
- 1 bay leaf
- 2 celery stalks, halved
- ¼ cup fresh basil, chopped
- 3 tablespoons homemade vegetable broth
- 2 tablespoons balsamic vinegar
- ¼ teaspoon Italian seasoning
- 2 tablespoons tomato paste

How to Prepare
1. In a pan of boiling water, add tomatoes and cook for about 1 minute.
2. Drain well and transfer into a bowl of ice water.
3. Let them cool. Remove the peel and seeds of the tomatoes.
4. Chop 2 tomatoes and set aside.
5. In a blender, add the remaining 8 tomatoes and pulse until a puree forms.
6. In a large pan, heat the oil over medium heat and sauté the carrots, celery, bell pepper, onion, and garlic, for about 5 minutes.
7. Add chopped tomatoes, tomato puree, and remaining all ingredients (except tomato paste) and bring to a boil.
8. Lower the heat to low and simmer for about 2 hours, stirring occasionally.
9. Stir in the tomato paste and simmer for about 2 hours more.
10. Discard the celery and bay leaf set aside to cool completely before serving.

Nutritional Values
- Calories 130
- Total Fat 7.6 g
- Saturated Fat 1.1 g
- Cholesterol 0 mg
- Sodium 60 mg
- Total Carbs 15.2 g
- Fiber 4 g
- Sugar 9 g
- Protein 3 g

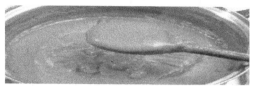

Mango BBQ Sauce

Preparation time: 15 minutes
Cooking time: 25 minutes
Total time: 40 minutes
Servings: 10

Ingredients
- ½ of Habanero pepper
- 1 cup mango, peeled, pitted, and chopped
- ½ tablespoon fresh ginger, chopped
- 2 tablespoons garlic, chopped
- ½ cup dates, pitted and chopped roughly
- 1 cup tomato sauce
- ¼ cup apple cider vinegar
- 2 teaspoons curry powder
- Salt and ground black pepper, to taste

How to Prepare
1. Preheat the broiler of the oven to high.
2. Arrange the Habanero pepper half onto a baking sheet, cut side down and broil for about 5–10 minutes.
3. Remove the pepper rom broiler and chop it.
4. In a pan, add pepper and remaining ingredients over medium-high heat and bring to a boil, stirring occasionally.
5. Lower the heat to medium and simmer for about 10 minutes, stirring occasionally.
6. Remove from heat and set aside to cool slightly.
7. In a food processor, add the mango mixture and pulse until smooth.
8. Set aside to cool completely before serving.

Nutritional Values
- Calories 48
- Total Fat 0.2 g
- Saturated Fat 0.1 g
- Cholesterol 0 mg
- Sodium 145 mg
- Total Carbs 11.7 g
- Fiber 1.6 g
- Sugar 9 g
- Protein 1 g

30-Day Meal Plan

Day 1
Breakfast: Pumpkin Porridge
Lunch: Chickpea Falafel Bowl
Dinner: Veggies Stew

Day 2
Breakfast: Fruity Tofu Smoothie
Lunch: Stuffed Sweet Potato
Dinner: Nut Roast Dinner

Day 3
Breakfast: Quinoa, Oats, & Seeds Porridge
Lunch: Tofu with Brussels Sprouts
Dinner: Beans with Salsa

Day 4
Breakfast: Savory Crepes
Lunch: Spicy Black Beans
Dinner: Rice Paella

Day 5
Breakfast: Green Smoothie Bowl
Lunch: Cauliflower with Peas
Dinner: Barley & Chickpea Soup

Day 6
Breakfast: Nuts, Seeds, & Coconut Granola
Lunch: Glazed Carrots
Dinner: 3-Bean Chili

Day 7
Breakfast: Fruity Muffins
Lunch: Chickpeas with Swiss Chard
Dinner: Barley & Lentil Stew

Day 8
Breakfast: Veggie Quiche
Lunch: Burgers with Mushroom Sauce
Dinner: Beans, Corn, & Salsa Chili

Day 9
Breakfast: Savory Crepes
Lunch: Lentil Falafel Bowl
Dinner: Nut Roast Dinner

Day 10
Breakfast: Pumpkin Porridge
Lunch: Baked Tofu
Dinner: Mixed Bean Soup

Day 11
Breakfast: Strawberry Shake
Lunch: Mushroom Curry
Dinner: Chili Corn Carne

Day 12
Breakfast: Barley Porridge
Lunch: Stuffed Avocado
Dinner: Beans & Quinoa with Veggies

Day 13
Breakfast: Banana Pancakes
Lunch: Baked Beans
Dinner: Tempeh with Bell Peppers

Day 14
Breakfast: Overnight Porridge
Lunch: 3-Veggie Combo
Dinner: Rice Paella

Day 15
Breakfast: Blueberry Waffles
Lunch: Banana Curry
Dinner: Bean & Pasta Stew

Day 16
Breakfast: Banana Pancakes
Lunch: Lentil Falafel Bowl
Dinner: Chickpea & Veggie Bake

Day 17
Breakfast: Overnight Porridge
Lunch: Buckwheat Burgers
Dinner: Rice & Lentil Casserole

Day 18
Breakfast: Veggie Omelet
Lunch: Rice & Tofu Salad
Dinner: Black-Eyed Peas Curry

Day 19
Breakfast: Green Smoothie Bowl
Lunch: Vegetarian Taco Bowl
Dinner: 3-Bean Chili

Day 20
Breakfast: Veggie Quiche
Lunch: Tofu with Peas
Dinner: Lentil Curry

Day 21
Breakfast: Fruity Muffins
Lunch: Tofu & Veggie Burgers
Dinner: Nut Roast Dinner

Day 22
Breakfast: Green Smoothie Bowl

Lunch: Burgers with Mushroom Sauce
Dinner: Bean & Lentil Stew
Day 23
Breakfast: Blueberry Waffles
Lunch: Pasta with Asparagus
Dinner: Chickpea & Pasta Curry
Day 24
Breakfast: Fruity Muffins
Lunch: Carrot Soup with tempeh
Dinner: Rice & Lentil Casserole
Day 25
Breakfast: Spinach & Tomato Omelet
Lunch: Chickpeas with Swiss Chard
Dinner: Veggie Stew
Day 26
Breakfast: Banana Pancakes
Lunch: Dried Fruit Squash
Dinner: Barley & Chickpea Soup
Day 27
Breakfast: Green Fruity Smoothie
Lunch: Couscous Stuffed Bell Peppers
Dinner: Tempeh with Bell Peppers
Day 28
Breakfast: Nuts, Seeds & Coconut Granola
Lunch: Buddha Bowl
Dinner: Chickpea & Pasta Curry
Day 29
Breakfast: Barley Porridge
Lunch: Glazed Carrots
Dinner: Barley & Lentil Stew
Day 30
Breakfast: Savory Crepes
Lunch: Farro Salad
Dinner: Lentil Soup

Cheap Shopping List

Vegetables:
- Onion (yellow, red, white, etc.)
- Garlic
- Fresh ginger
- Tomato
- Carrot
- Sweet potato
- Zucchini
- Eggplant
- Celery stalks
- Fresh mushrooms (shiitake, cremini, button, etc.)
- Broccoli
- Cauliflower
- Cabbage (purple, green, Napa, Bok Choy, etc.)
- Green peas
- Asparagus
- Bell peppers (red, yellow, green, orange)
- Pumpkin
- Asparagus
- Green beans
- Brussels sprouts
- Beets
- Leafy greens (spinach, kale, collard greens, Swiss chard, etc.)
- Cucumbers
- Radishes
- Lemons
- Limes
- Lettuce (Romaine, endive, butter head, loose-leaf, etc.)
- Peppers (Habanero, jalapeño, Serrano, etc.)
- Fresh herbs (cilantro, parsley, rosemary, thyme, oregano, basil, etc.)

Fruit
- Avocados
- Apples
- Pears
- Oranges
- Grapes
- Berries (strawberries, blueberries, raspberries, etc.)
- Kiwi
- Melons (cantaloupe, watermelon, honeydew, etc.)
- Pineapple
- Mango
- Peach
- Bananas

Grains, Beans, & Legumes
- Beans (Chickpeas, Cannellini beans, kidney beans, Great Northern beans, Pinto beans, Black beans, etc.)

- Legumes (lentils, black-eyed peas, split peas, etc.)
- Oats (old-fashioned oats, rolled oats, quick oats, etc.)
- Barley
- Bulgur wheat
- Quinoa
- Brown rice
- Whole-wheat pasta
- Wild rice
- Farro
- Couscous
- Millet

Seasonings & Spices

- Salt
- Black pepper
- Cinnamon
- Nutmeg
- Cardamom
- Cumin
- Coriander
- Garlic powder
- Onion powder
- Dried herbs (parsley, rosemary, thyme, basil, oregano, etc.)
- Turmeric
- Curry powder
- Paprika
- Cayenne pepper
- Red chili powder
- Red pepper flakes
- Bay leaves
- Italian seasoning

Extras

- Non-dairy milk (almond milk, coconut milk, hemp milk, soymilk, cashew milk, etc.)
- Nut butter (cashew, almond, peanut butter, etc.)
- Cooking oils (olive, vegetable, canola, coconut oil, sesame oil, etc.)
- Flours (whole-wheat, almond, coconut, chickpea flour, arrowroot flour, etc.)
- Seeds (hemp, pumpkin, sunflower, flax, chia, sesame seeds, etc.)
- Nuts (pistachios, almonds, walnuts, pecan, hazelnuts, cashews, etc.)
- Dried fruit (raisins, dried cherries, dried cranberries, figs, apricots, dates, etc.)
- Sauces (soy sauce, Sriracha, hot pepper sauce, Worcestershire sauce, etc.)
- Sweeteners (maple syrup, unsweetened applesauce, etc.)
- Vinegars (balsamic, apple cider, white wine vinegar, etc.)
- Tomato based products (sugar-free tomato paste, tomato puree, tomato sauce, salsa, etc.)
- Meat-free proteins (tofu, tempeh, etc.)
- Cornstarch
- Baking powder
- Baking soda
- Coconut flakes
- Vegan chocolate chips
- Unsweetened vegan protein powder
- Cacao powder
- Coffee powder
- Tahini
- Hummus
- Mustard
- Vanilla extract
- Nutritional yeast

CPSIA information can be obtained
at www.ICGtesting.com
Printed in the USA
LVHW060509080221
678690LV00006B/45